A Gastroenterologist's Guide to Gut Health

A Gastroenterologist's Guide to Gut Health

Everything You Need to Know about Colonoscopy, Digestive Diseases, and Healthy Eating

David M. Novick, MD

ROWMAN & LITTLEFIELD
Lanham • Boulder • New York • London

Disclaimer

This book contains general medical information. It is not intended to provide any recommendations or advice to a specific individual and should not be used for this purpose. While the author has made his best effort to provide reliable and accurate information, no warranty or guarantee is made regarding any statement in this book. The medical statements in this book are the opinion of the author and do not necessarily represent the opinions of the medical community. The medical information presented should not be considered as a complete or comprehensive discussion of the subject. All readers should discuss their own health care with their primary or specialist physicians or both. For all medications, the package insert should be reviewed for the correct use, drug interactions, and side effects, as well as any other question concerning the medication.

Medical science is an evolving and rapidly-changing field, and advances in medical knowledge, procedures, medical devices, and drug therapy may occur at any time. The standard of care for a given issue may have changed since the publication of this book. Again, the reader is advised to discuss any medical questions with, and obtain medical advice from, his or her personal physician.

The author disclaims any responsibility for any action, or the results of any action, based on the information provided herein.

All images by David M. Novick are © 2016 by Archaeopteryx Media LLC.

Published by Rowman & Littlefield
A wholly owned subsidary of The Rowman & Littlefield Publishing Group, Inc.
4501 Forbes Boulevard, Suite 200, Lanham, Maryland 20706
www.rowman.com

Unit A, Whitacre Mews, 26-34 Stannary Street, London SE11 4AB

British Library Cataloguing in Publication Information Available

Library of Congress Cataloging-in-Publication Data

Names: Novick, David M., 1948– author.
Title: A gastroenterologist's guide to gut health : everything you need to
    know about colonoscopy, digestive diseases, and healthy eating / David M.
    Novick.
Description: Lanham : Rowman & Littlefield, [2017] | Includes bibliographical
    references and index.
Identifiers: LCCN 2016040787 (print) | LCCN 2016042084 (ebook) | ISBN
    9781442271982 (cloth) | ISBN 9781442271999 (ebook)
Subjects: LCSH: Gastrointestinal system—Diseases—Popular works. |
    Gastrointestinal system—Diseases—Diet therapy.
Classification: LCC RC806 .N68 2017 (print) | LCC RC806 (ebook) | DDC
    616.3/3—dc23
LC record available at https://lccn.loc.gov/2016040787

♾™ The paper used in this publication meets the minimum requirements of
American National Standard for Information Sciences—Permanence of Paper
for Printed Library Materials, ANSI/NISO Z39.48-1992.

Printed in the United States of America

For Jane

Contents

Introduction

People want accurate medical information. Medical issues increasingly compete with other stories for top positions in the news media. We live in an information age, but how can people be sure that what they get is accurate, let alone understandable? I wrote this book to address that need.

Some have asked why write a book on gut health when anyone can get plenty of medical information on the Internet. There are three main problems with that widespread practice. First, in your reading, you could easily misdiagnose yourself, leading to unnecessary worry and poor decision making. For example, you might read about adverse effects, complications, or death in medical conditions that you do not have. Second, you might find information that is false or misleading. Today I read an online story with beautiful graphics, concerning a "new cancer treatment," that was supposedly a breakthrough, based on a single abstract from a research meeting (abstracts are short, preliminary communications that are not reviewed by peers in the scientific community). Third, you might end up on a reliable website that is too complex and not understandable without significant necessary background information, leading to misconceptions that you and your doctor will need to address.

This book intends to give you the basic information you need to understand the common problems of the gastrointestinal (GI) tract. A glossary in the back explains the medical terms. You will also find a helpful list of recommended books and websites.

For the record, this book started as the medical background for a collection of GI humor. As I was writing it, I realized that there might be a need to provide more information to the patient, to help him or her learn more about the GI symptoms, the procedures, and the treatments that may be required.

In addition to gaining a better understanding, this may help lessen some of the anxiety for the patient. The humor book is still awaiting the signal to go. Please check my website, www.drdavidnovick.com, for status updates.

Is there a need for a book about gut health? Let's look at some numbers. Colonoscopy is the most effective method for screening and preventing colon cancer, and it is estimated that fourteen million colonoscopies are performed in the United States each year. Despite this large number, despite marketing campaigns by colon cancer charities, hospitals, and doctors, and despite frequent jokes by late-night comedians, the American Cancer Society estimates that there will still be 134,490 new cases of colon cancer in the United States in 2016, and 49,190 deaths from this disease.[1] Similar numbers, or higher, have been seen in preceding years. That's almost as many deaths **every year** as occurred among Americans in the entire Vietnam War. The costs of colon cancer treatment are expected to reach $15–20 billion annually by 2020.[2] Because too many people do not undergo colon cancer screening, one of the aims of this book is to promote colon cancer screening and empower people to make an educated decision about colonoscopy or alternative screening methods.

What about other GI diseases?

- Irritable bowel syndrome is the most common GI disease and is thought to affect 10–15 percent of the adult population.[3] It is most common in women under age forty-five and is second only to the common cold in causing days missed from work.
- Crohn's disease and ulcerative colitis (collectively known as inflammatory bowel disease) together affect between 1 and 1.3 million persons in the United States.[4]
- Diverticulosis is found in 40–60 percent of people in the United States over age sixty.[5]
- About 60 million people in the United States have occasional heartburn (acid reflux, gastroesophageal reflux), and 15 million have heartburn every day.[6]

This book aims to give you useful and reliable information on these and many other GI conditions, based on the advice that I give to patients every day. The illustrations are typical of those seen in my medical practice. Please note:

- This is not a medical textbook and cannot cover every disease or situation.
- This book should not replace the advice of your personal physician (please see the disclaimers), but it is the only book that covers the most

common GI problems and tells you what your gastroenterologist wants you to know.

- Although names of products (including brand names) are mentioned when necessary, I am not endorsing any product or brand.
- Medical literature uses the term "colorectal cancer" to include colon and rectal cancer. For simplicity, I use "colon cancer" to denote both of these.
- Although gastroenterologists are the focus of this book, some qualified surgeons also perform GI procedures, including colonoscopy.

Gut health is a relatively new yet popular term. What exactly is gut health? Most people tend to think of gut health as the absence of the wide variety of possible GI symptoms. Traditional medical practice conducts an evaluation and treatment of such symptoms and the underlying diseases that cause them. At the same time, many will agree that health, including gut health, is more than merely the absence of symptoms or disease, and that prevention is better than treatment. The World Health Organization adopted a positive definition of health in 1946 that included a sense of physical, mental, and social well-being.[7]

In the spirit of generating a positive definition of gut health for 2017, I suggest that gut health is the absence of GI symptoms, the effective treatment of GI symptoms and diseases using evidence-based methods, use of prevention techniques, and healthy eating. Maintenance of gut health today involves three major efforts. First, prevention of GI disorders whenever possible is critical. Getting a colonoscopy at the appropriate age will go a long way toward preventing colon cancer and is the single most important thing that a healthy person can do to maintain gut health (see chapters 1–7). Although more research is needed in preventing other GI diseases, preventive measures you can take now include limiting pancreatitis (chapter 16) and liver cirrhosis (chapter 18) by avoiding excessive alcohol use. You can also prevent hepatitis C (chapter 17) by not misusing opioids or other drugs intravenously and by effectively treating opioid addiction. Second, treating GI diseases with the most effective approaches is an essential component of gut health. Such treatment will often involve medications which may have significant toxicity, and gut health will be maximized by the careful use of these agents. Third, promoting healthy eating is a major challenge of our time. Recent estimates published in 2016 suggest that two billion people worldwide are overweight and 600 million are obese.[8] This obesity epidemic is expected to lead to massive increases in the numbers of people with heart disease, diabetes mellitus, hypertension, and liver cirrhosis.[9] Chapter 19 discusses the principles of healthy eating.

A more limited view of gut health is found in many articles on gut health today, especially those found on the Internet; these articles point to two abnormalities that may harm gut health.[10-12] First, the normal set of microorganisms, numbering in the trillions, that inhabit the intestinal tract (the microbiome, discussed in chapter 19) can become altered and depleted by factors that are common in today's lifestyle: unhealthy diets, chemicals, antibiotics, other medications, stress, and infections. These same factors may cause damage to the intestinal barrier, i.e., the intestinal wall, which is the barrier between the intestinal contents and the body. The damaged intestinal barrier could become more permeable and allow bacteria, chemicals, or large molecules from food to enter the bloodstream, a situation referred to as "leaky gut syndrome." These foreign substances are attacked by the immune system, and the resulting immunologic reactions are proposed to lead to many GI and non-GI diseases, especially autoimmune diseases (see glossary). The microbiome and intestinal barrier can be restored by probiotics (see chapter 19), a healthy diet, use of supplements, adding hydrochloric acid or acidic foods, and avoiding the causative factors listed above.

While the above narrative has helped raise consciousness about healthy living and prevention, it is based on assumptions and incomplete knowledge. The microbiome is of immense importance, but our knowledge of it is in its infancy. There are microorganisms living in our intestines that have not been identified and cannot be grown in laboratory cultures.[13] Probiotics and fermentable foods (see chapters 9 and 19) may help restore the microbiome, but reliable information on which ones, how much, and for how long is lacking. The intestinal barrier is important, but we don't know if abnormalities in it are a cause or a result of disease; nor do we have clinically significant information on how to measure barrier function and how to treat barrier dysfunction.[14,15] Finally, by excluding pharmaceutical therapeutics from the recommendations, this narrative may harm gut health by causing people to eschew beneficial therapies.

When I was in medical school, GI courses began with the esophagus and progressed downward. Here, I will break with tradition and start with colonoscopy and colon cancer prevention, since this is why most people visit a gastroenterologist for the first time.

THE GASTROINTESTINAL TRACT

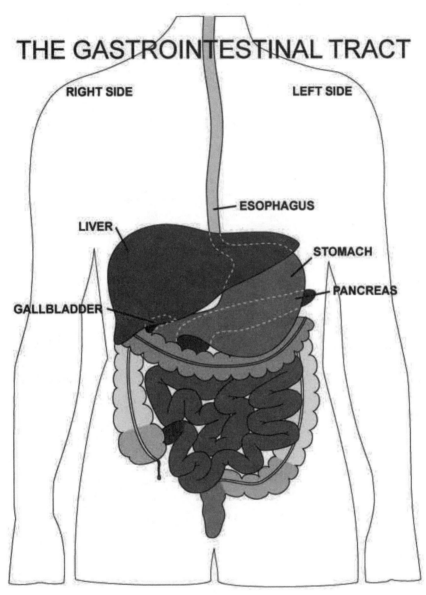

RIGHT SIDE

LEFT SIDE

ESOPHAGUS

LIVER

STOMACH

PANCREAS

GALLBLADDER

Diagram 1.   The gastrointestinal tract. Source: Ellyn Miller, *Gastrointestinal Tract*, May 2014. © Archaeopteryx Media LLC.

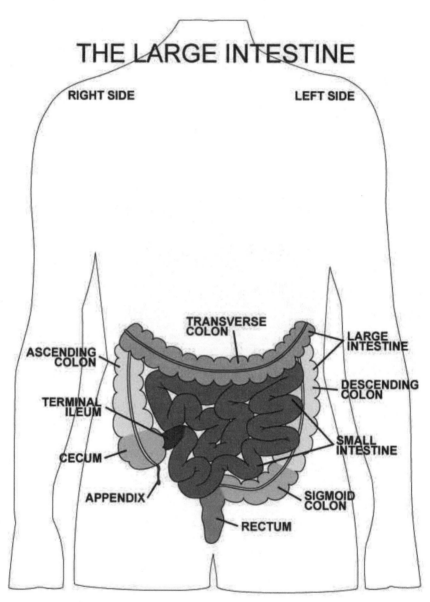

THE LARGE INTESTINE

RIGHT SIDE   LEFT SIDE

TRANSVERSE COLON

LARGE INTESTINE

ASCENDING COLON

DESCENDING COLON

TERMINAL ILEUM

SMALL INTESTINE

CECUM

APPENDIX

SIGMOID COLON

RECTUM

Diagram 2. The large intestine. Source: Ellyn Miller, *Large Intestine*, May 2014. ©
Archaeopteryx Media LLC.

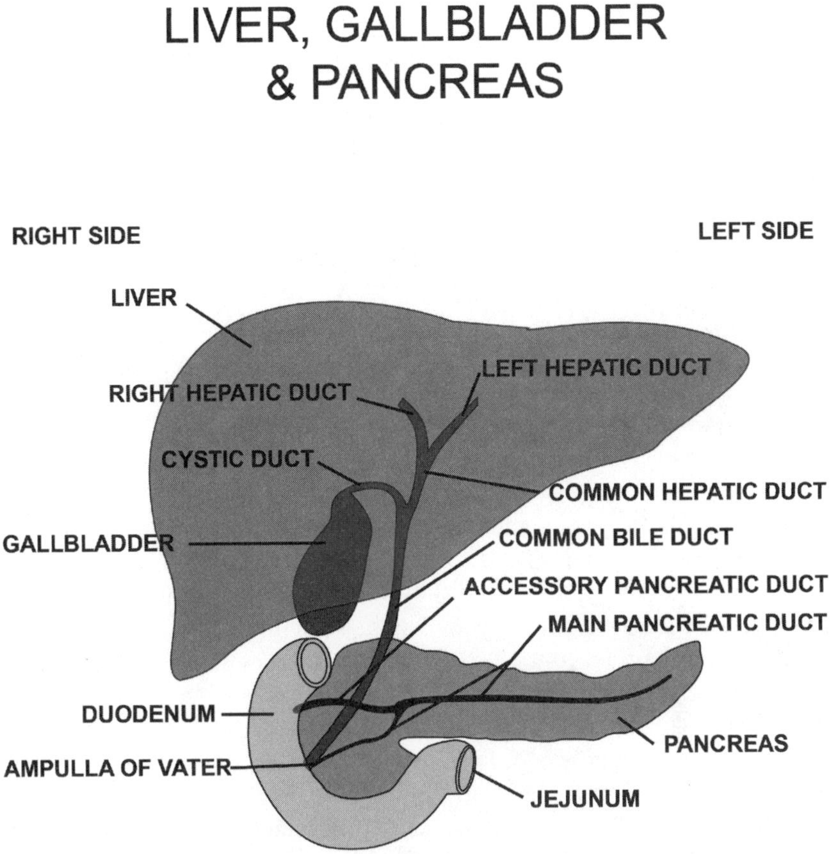

LIVER, GALLBLADDER & PANCREAS

Diagram 3.   The liver, gallbladder, and pancreas. Source: Shannon Simpson, *Liver, Gallbladder, Pancreas*, June 2016. © Archaeopteryx Media LLC.

1

Preparing for Colonoscopy

Colonoscopy is the examination of the colon, or large intestine, using a long flexible scope (figure 1.1). The scope makes possible detailed viewing, high-resolution photography, and removal of polyps (growths) or tissue for analysis (biopsy). Successful colonoscopy requires a high-quality "bowel prep," in which laxatives are taken to clear the fecal matter, or stool, from the colon so that important details can be seen. Colonoscopy is done at an outpatient center or hospital and is the primary method of colon cancer screening in use today, and the most accurate. For other methods, see chapter 6, "Colonoscopy: Risks, Alternatives, and Barriers."

Colonoscopy is a potentially life-saving procedure. It can greatly reduce your odds of getting colon cancer. The first four chapters will take you through the steps of colonoscopy from the beginning to end, so you will know exactly what to expect.

The first step in a successful medical procedure such as colonoscopy is making the decision to do it. Many people are reluctant to have a colonoscopy because of the need for a bowel prep, a fear of pain, or a loss of control. All of these concerns should be discussed with your doctor. He or she can review the risks (discussed in chapter 6), benefits, and prep options and address any special issues you may have. Details on the reasons why people refuse a colonoscopy, and my thoughts on overcoming them, are also found in chapter 6.

In addition to colon cancer screening, colonoscopy is also very useful for evaluation of gastrointestinal bleeding, diarrhea, constipation, change in bowel habits, abdominal pain, and abnormal imaging studies (X-ray or CT scan).

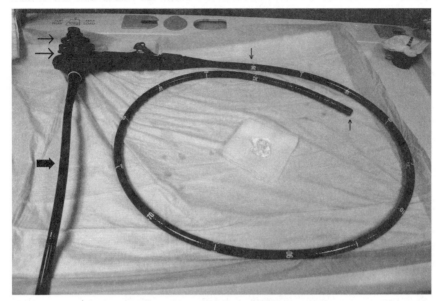

Figure 1.1.   The colonoscope. Arrows, starting from the far right and proceeding clockwise: 1. The tip; the first part inserted into the patient. 2. Tube that connects the scope to the power source. 3 (upper). Dial that turns the tip right or left. 4. (lower). Dial that turns the tip up or down. Rotation up to 180° is possible. 5. Last measured insertion point, 160 cm from tip.
Source: David M. Novick, *The Colonoscope,* July 2016.

Once you make the decision to have a colonoscopy, you will be given detailed instructions on diet, medications, and how and when to take your bowel prep. You really do need to have your colon cleaned out well so your doctor can see the fine details. Even a small quantity of retained stool can obscure polyps, bleeding sites, abnormal blood vessels, or areas of inflammation. Figure 1.2 shows the normal colon with tiny blood vessels clearly seen; this is the degree of detail that your doctor needs to see.

The traditional bowel prep for colonoscopy involves drinking up to a gallon of solution to flush out the entire accumulation of stool that is stored in the colon. Recently, smaller-volume prep solutions have been introduced. It is really important to drink extra fluids of various types on the day before your procedure, especially before starting the prep solution, in order to remain well hydrated. Your physician will give you a list of the liquids that are not allowed (see box on the following page). You should not have any solid food on the day before your colonoscopy.

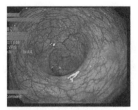 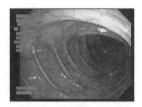 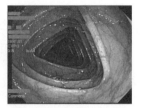

Figure 1.2. Three normal views of parts of the colon. Left: rectum. Center: descending colon. Right: transverse colon. Triangular folds are common in this area. Note the detailed blood vessels in all three images, a typical feature of the lining of the normal large intestine.

Source: David M. Novick, *Rectum,* July 2016.

THE BOWEL PREP

Regarding the bowel prep, please read the instructions from your physician carefully, preferably one week before your procedure. If you wait until the night before, your procedure will not happen! You have definitely waited too long. Most preps include the following elements:

- **Seven days before colonoscopy**: Do not eat any foods containing the fat substitute olestra, also known as Olean, and stop taking iron supplements.
- **Three days before colonoscopy**: Do not eat high-fiber foods, including fruits, vegetables, salads, nuts, and seeds.
- **One day before colonoscopy**: Start a clear liquid diet and eat no solid foods.

CLEAR LIQUIDS FOR COLONOSCOPY PREP

- Clear fruit juice
- White grape juice
- Sports drinks—Lower-calorie items preferred
- Clear soup, broth, or bouillon
- Water
- Tea or coffee—**No cream**
- Hard candies
- Jell-O or popsicles
- Carbonated beverages not recommended unless "flat"
- **Nothing red or purple**
- **No alcohol**

For Best Results, Use a Variety of These

Red or purple liquids should be avoided as they may resemble blood.

You will usually start the prep in the early evening of the day before the colonoscopy. All preps contain some type of liquid designed to clean out your colon. It is important to drink all of it. Most preps are given in two parts: one part in the early evening and the other in the early morning. The exact times will depend on the time of your procedure.

Example: Your arrival time for colonoscopy is at 8:00 AM, and your prep is with polyethylene glycol (PEG) solution (MiraLAX, GlycoLax, and others). Starting at 6:00 PM the evening before, you will take seventeen grams of powder mixed in eight ounces of clear liquid every fifteen minutes for a total of seven doses. The seven doses should be completed in two hours.

Then, at 1:00 AM, you will start the second part, another seven doses of the PEG solution as described above. These seven doses should also be completed in two hours, e.g., at 3:00 AM, which is five hours before your arrival time.

Splitting the dose of the prep in this way results in much better clean-outs, allowing your gastroenterologist to see what needs to be seen. Split-dose preps are also easier to tolerate than drinking the entire volume at once. You should complete all of your laxatives by three to five hours before your colonoscopy.[1] After that, you should have nothing by mouth, except if you take certain critical medications mentioned below. **People with diabetes will be given special instructions**. It is very important to discuss any questions about medications with your physician.

Table 1.1 shows prep solutions in current use. Although brand names are shown, I am not endorsing any particular brand. Insurance coverage for the more expensive preps is variable.

At some point during the prep, you should start to pass clear liquid. This is the intended result, but do not stop the prep at that point. Continue drinking until it is all gone. Your prep instructions may also contain tablets such as bisacodyl, a laxative, or simethicone, to break up gas bubbles. Take these as instructed.

After the drinking is done:

- Strictly nothing by mouth until your procedure is complete.
- Do not chew gum.
- Exception: If you take medicine for your heart, high blood pressure, or seizures, take these with a small sip of water close to your usual time, but at least two hours before your procedure.

Table 1.1. Bowel Preps in Common Use

Prep	Main Ingredient	Volume (Part 1)	Volume (Part 2)	Cost*	Comments
MiraLAX, GlycoLax, or others	Polyethylene glycol (PEG)	8 oz. for 7 doses (56 oz.)	Same as Part 1	+	Comes as powder; mix with clear liquid of your choice. Can cause low sodium in patients over 70.
GoLYTELY, NuLYTELY, or others	PEG and electrolytes	8 oz. for 8 doses (64 oz.)	Same as Part 1	+	Largest volume
MoviPrep	PEG and electrolytes	8 oz. for 4 doses (32 oz.) followed by 16 oz. clear liquid (total 48 oz.)	Same as Part 1	++++	
SUPREP	Sodium sulfate and electrolytes	16 oz. followed by 32 oz. clear liquid (48 oz.)	Same as Part 1	++++	Most of the volume is the clear liquid of your choice.
PREPOPIK	Sodium picosulfate, magnesium oxide, and citric acid	5 oz. followed by 8 oz. clear liquid for 5 doses (45 oz.)	Same as Part 1	++++	

*Cost: + = $1–30, ++++ = $91–120.

Source: www.goodrx.com.

URGENT QUESTION

Q. What if I have nausea or vomiting while drinking the prep?

A. Stop and wait one hour; then resume the prep and finish it. If you still cannot drink it, call your doctor for further instructions. Often an alternative prep is recommended, such as a ten-ounce bottle of magnesium citrate. Do not take magnesium citrate if you have kidney disease. (It's OK if you have a history of kidney stones.)

Occasionally, bowel preps are inadequate despite your having followed all of the instructions. There is an increased risk for an inadequate bowel prep in people with the following medical conditions: history of previous inadequate prep, constipation, medications such as opioids that are constipating, diabetes mellitus, and obesity. Poor preps are also increased in people who have a long wait between scheduling and the procedure date. A two-day prep will be needed for a subsequent colonoscopy when the initial prep is inadequate.

Two final notes about preps:

- Do not use any laxative containing sodium phosphate for cleansing for colonoscopy. These may cause kidney damage.
- Polyethylene glycol is NOT antifreeze. Antifreezes may contain ethylene glycol and propylene glycol, among other compounds.

Since you will almost certainly be sedated during your procedure, you will not be permitted to drive afterward and until the following day. Although you might feel fine, your reflexes will not be as quick as normal in the event of an accident. You should make no plans until the next day. After the procedure, you may eat at home but may not go to a restaurant, as you might lose your balance because of the sedation and injure yourself. You should not go out to any event, such as a graduation or a concert.

Since you cannot drive after your procedure, you will need a driver. A few notes about drivers:

- Make sure your driver has blocked off the time in his or her schedule. Medical procedures cannot be rushed and do not always finish on time. It can be a problem if your driver is eager to leave before you are ready.
- You may NOT take a taxi if you are alone. A taxi driver will not escort you into your home and help you get settled. Remember, there will still be sedative in your body after the procedure.
- You may take a cab if you are accompanied by a competent adult. This person should ensure that you are safely ensconced in your home.
- In the rare case that your procedure is done without sedation, you may drive or take a cab home on your own. Even then, having a companion with you is optimal.

After you arrive at the endoscopy unit or hospital, your medical history will be reviewed and vital signs will be checked. A nurse will review your medications and pharmacy information. You will change into a gown that opens in the back, and you will have a brief physical examination. A small needle will be inserted into a vein in your arm for intravenous access.

You will sign a consent form for the procedure itself, for the anesthesia, or for the lack of anesthesia if you do not wish to be sedated. You will also sign a form indicating that you understand that if you have taken aspirin, Plavix, or Coumadin (anticoagulants, or "blood thinners") recently, you might bleed if a biopsy is done or a polyp is removed.

A nurse, endoscopy technician, or medical assistant will answer any questions you may have, and you are now ready for your procedure.

TAKE-HOME MESSAGES

- Colon cancer is the third most common cause of cancer death in men and women in the United States. Before the widespread use of screening colonoscopy, colon cancer was the second leading cause.
- Most cases of colon cancer can be prevented by screening, usually by colonoscopy. See chapter 5, "The Evidence, Quality Issues, and Surveillance Intervals" for details and chapter 6 for alternatives to colonoscopy.
- Read your prep instructions carefully five to seven days before your procedure. During your prep, you should start passing clear liquid. If the prep is not working, or if you have other problems, call your doctor.
- You must have someone to drive you home unless your procedure is without sedation. You should have no other plans for the rest of the day.
- Ask questions. Don't be embarrassed to ask. Any question is OK.

2

Sedation and Anesthesia

There are two methods of sedation in use today for colonoscopy or upper GI endoscopy: conscious sedation or total IV anesthesia (TIVA). Conscious sedation (also known as moderate sedation or twilight sleep) is ordered by the gastroenterologist performing the procedure and administered by a nurse intravenously in repeated small doses before and during the procedure as needed. Conscious sedation is usually a combination of an analgesic (pain medication) and a sedative. Fentanyl is commonly used for analgesia, and midazolam (Versed) or diazepam (Valium) for sedation. The dose is individualized such that the patient is lightly sleeping, but at least partially responsive, so that if the nurse speaks loudly she or he will be heard. Although patients receiving conscious sedation are not "completely out," they almost always have no memory of the procedure since brief amnesia is a side effect of midazolam.

TIVA is given by an anesthesiologist or nurse anesthetist, and it provides a deeper sedation that requires more careful monitoring. Propofol is the medication most commonly used. It may be used alone or combined with other agents such as fentanyl or midazolam. Because propofol has a rapid onset and also wears off very quickly, its use requires constant monitoring by an anesthesiologist (who is a medical doctor) or a certified nurse anesthetist. The need for an additional person increases the cost of the procedure. In some states, other health professionals with special training may administer this drug. Propofol has a milky white appearance and is often referred to as "The Milk of Amnesia" or "The Milk of Anesthesia," an obvious play on words on the laxative Milk of Magnesia. It is a very effective anesthetic and provides a deeper level of anesthesia than conscious sedation. After receiving it, patients wake up feeling like they have had a very refreshing sleep.

PROPOFOL AND MICHAEL JACKSON

Propofol received great notoriety when Michael Jackson died on June 25, 2009, after receiving the drug *at home, without proper monitoring.*[1-4] He also received several benzodiazepines (the class of drugs that includes midazolam and diazepam as mentioned previously, as well as several commonly prescribed sedatives). The doctor was convicted of involuntary manslaughter.[5-7] For the next few months, many patients were reluctant to receive this drug, but such concerns were usually resolved after explaining that the drug is safe when administered by a trained professional in an accredited ambulatory surgery unit or hospital. More recently, there have been increased requests for propofol, probably as a result of enhanced public awareness that it is an excellent medication when used properly.

Many factors influence the decision on which type of anesthesia to use in GI procedures. TIVA is preferred in patients with a history of regular use of narcotic (opioid) pain medications, sedatives such as benzodiazepines, or past/ongoing heavy alcohol use. Conscious sedation is likely to be ineffective in such patients. Also, patients with significant heart or lung disease (such as coronary artery disease with stents, emphysema, or sleep apnea) benefit from the close monitoring by the anesthesiologist or nurse anesthetist. In many GI practices, propofol is used in most patients, even those without specific risk factors, because of its effectiveness and convenience. If the patient wants "to be totally out," TIVA is more likely to be effective; if he or she fears total loss of control, conscious sedation may be preferred. The decision on the type of anesthesia is best based on the individual needs of the patient. Table 2.1 summarizes the key features of both types.

Table 2.1.   Comparison of Conscious Sedation and Total IV Anesthesia

	Conscious Sedation	*Total IV Anesthesia (TIVA)*
Onset*	Gradual	Rapid
Offset*	Gradual	Rapid
Administered by . . .	Nurse, per doctor's orders	Anesthesiologist
	Gastroenterologist	Certified Nurse Anesthetist (CRNA)
Medication most commonly used	Fentanyl and midazolam (Versed)	Propofol
Depth of sedation	++	++++
Amnesic effect**	++++	0 or +
Cost***	+	+++

* Individual results may vary. Regardless of the rapidity of the offset, you may not drive until the next day.
** Forgetfulness of the time when the drug is active, seen with midazolam (Versed).
*** There will be an additional fee for the anesthesiologist or CRNA.

Both types of anesthesia used in endoscopic procedures today are safe and effective. Because changes in heart rate, blood pressure, and oxygen tension may occur with either, close monitoring is mandatory.

Patients worry that when sedated they will reveal personal or embarrassing details, but this is virtually never the case. Regardless of whether conscious sedation or TIVA is used, most people just go to sleep—they say less and less as they get sleepier and sleepier. Rarely, patients speak briefly during their procedures.

Patients receiving TIVA or conscious sedation require close monitoring. Until recently, standard monitoring consisted of measuring heart rate and oxygen saturation continuously, and blood pressure intermittently, all by machine. Cardiac rhythm was viewed on the monitor, similar to an electrocardiogram (top panel on the machine in figure 2.1), and a printout could be done if needed. Newer monitoring devices (figure 2.1) measure carbon dioxide (CO_2) levels and respiratory rate as well.

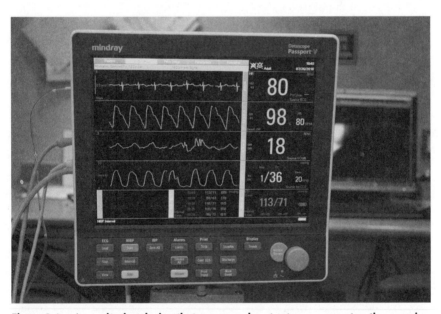

Figure 2.1.   A monitoring device that measures heart rate, oxygen saturation, respiratory rate, carbon dioxide, and blood pressure.

Source: David M. Novick, *CO_2 Monitor,* July 2016.

CASE REPORT: AMAZING ADVANCES IN TECHNOLOGY

Dr. Marks, a gastroenterologist, and Dr. Farra, an anesthesiologist (not their real names), were talking about the new monitors with special nasal cannulas for CO_2 monitoring. Dr. Marks was excited to try this new technology and see how it would contribute to patient care. The conversation moved to how far medicine has advanced. Dr. Farra had gone to medical school in India, and during her studies she was required to spend six months working in outlying rural areas. "In some areas, there was no hospital for more than a hundred miles," she recounted. "The medical team had to set up camp in an open area. For surgery, ether was used for anesthesia. A gauze pad was soaked with ether and placed over the patient's nose and mouth. The doctors would then administer the ether using an aluminum soft drink can which rested on a small table near the patient's head. The can had two openings on top. A tube resembling a straw ran from one of the openings to the patient's nose and a cotton swab was gently placed in the other opening. If they could see this cotton swab moving up and down, they knew that the patient was breathing!" She paused, then added, "The changes in medical technology just during my career are truly breathtaking."

TAKE-HOME MESSAGES

- Anesthesia for GI procedures is safe and effective.
- Propofol is a potent drug that is administered intravenously by an anesthesiologist or nurse anesthetist (some states may allow other trained personnel to give propofol).
- Propofol has a rapid onset and wears off quickly. It requires close monitoring.
- The cost of propofol is greater than that of conscious sedation because of the need for an additional health care professional.
- Conscious sedation, usually consisting of fentanyl and Versed, is given by a nurse per orders from the doctor doing the procedure.
- The decision on type of anesthesia is best individualized. The patient who wants to be "completely out" may be best managed with propofol, whereas one that is anxious about loss of control may be better off with conscious sedation.
- People almost never say anything embarrassing while sedated. The rare exceptions will be forgotten once awake. All medical staff are obligated to adhere to high standards of confidentiality. What happens in the procedure room stays in the procedure room (case reports in this book are included with written consent of the patient or with details changed and no identifiers).

3

The Colonoscopy

Once you are wheeled into the room where the procedure will be done, a last-minute verification will be carried out. This protocol is called a "time out" and it is based on quality control procedures developed in the airline industry. The doctor, nurse, anesthesiologist or nurse anesthetist (if any), and you will confirm your name, date of birth, the name of the doctor, and the procedure to be done. This is to confirm that the right procedure is done on the right patient. If all are in agreement, the sedation and procedure can begin.

The nurse will position you on your left side and will check that you have removed your underpants. You would be surprised how many people forget this last, yet critical step.

After the sedation has been initiated, the GI doctor will perform a rectal examination with a gloved finger and plenty of surgical lubricant, and then will insert the scope into the rectum, also with generous lubrication. The scope will be advanced into the colon while the image is viewed on a monitor on the other side of the patient. Air is pumped in through the scope in order to inflate the colon and allow better visualization. Normally in the colon, twists and turns are encountered. Gastroenterologists have several ways of negotiating these angles, such as gentle suctioning, pressure on the abdomen applied by the nurse, or pulling back on the scope to uncoil any loops in the scope.

Polyps, or growths, may be encountered at any point during the colonoscopy (figure 3.1). Details on the types of polyps, along with their cause and significance, are found in chapter 4, "Recovery after Colonoscopy"; chapter 5, "Putting Colonoscopy in Perspective: The Evidence, Quality Issues, and Surveillance Intervals"; and in the glossary. While some polyps are obvious, others may be very subtle. Careful attention to detail is important to ensure a high-quality colonoscopy (see chapter 5 for what constitutes a high-quality exam).

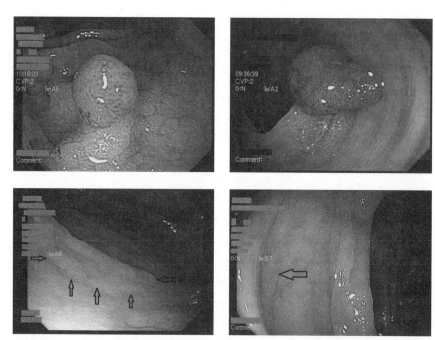

Figure 3.1.   Colon polyps. Upper left: An adenoma, a type of polyp that is potentially precancerous. Upper right: A high-risk adenoma because of its large size. Lower left: A very flat polyp, with the border shown by the arrows. This polyp was a sessile serrated adenoma. Lower right: A very small adenomatous polyp that was covered by a fold until just before the picture was taken. See also chapter 4, chapter 5, and the glossary.
Source: David M. Novick, *Colon Adenoma,* July 2016.

While carefully looking for any polyps or any other abnormalities, a major goal of the initial phase of the colonoscopy is the advancing of the scope to the cecum, the farthest point that the scope can reach in the large intestine. The cecum is located very low in the abdomen on the right side, close to the right hip bone. Entering the cecum means that the examination is complete. There are three important landmarks that will confirm that the cecum has been reached (figures 3.2 and 3.3): the ileocecal valve (a thick fold that serves as a doorway from the small intestine to the colon), the appendiceal orifice (opening to the appendix), and the terminal ileum (last part of the small intestine). The appendiceal orifice is seen even if the patient no longer has an appendix. A high-quality colonoscopy will include documentation of viewing at least two of these three landmarks.

Another way of knowing that the cecum has been reached is seeing the light from the scope shining through the skin in the right lower abdomen. The light can sometimes be obvious, but at other times only a trace of an orange glow is seen around a fingertip when pressed firmly against the abdominal

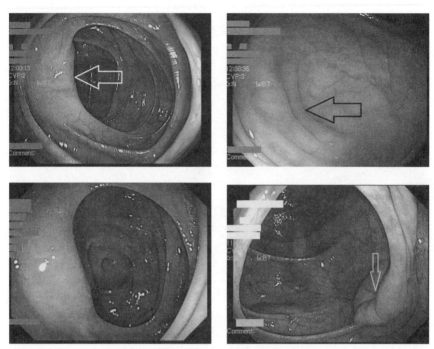

Figure 3.2. Normal anatomy of the cecum, ileocecal valve, and appendiceal orifice (opening to the appendix). The ileocecal valve and appendiceal orifice are important landmarks in colonoscopy. Upper left: The view as the scope approaches the cecum. The thick fold on the left (arrow) is the ileocecal valve, which connects the small and large intestine, usually on the back side of the valve. Upper right: As the scope is advanced farther, the crescent-shaped fold of the appendiceal orifice, or opening to the appendix (arrow), is seen. Lower left: The ileocecal valve on the left and the appendiceal orifice in the center are seen in the same image, showing their relationship. Lower right: The ileocecal valve is positioned such that the opening to the small intestine (arrow) is seen.
Source: David M. Novick, *Ileocecal Valve,* July 2016.

wall. In some patients, getting to the cecum can be challenging, even for an experienced gastroenterologist. There are many reasons why the cecum can be hard to reach: a long and tortuous colon, surgical adhesions (scar tissue from previous surgery), and enlargement of other intra-abdominal organs such as the spleen or uterus.

Once the cecum is reached and the landmarks are identified, the gastroenterologist will gradually remove the scope, using a slow, circular motion to look for polyps and any other abnormalities. When looking for polyps, the gastroenterologist carefully searches behind folds to locate as many as possible. Smaller polyps are painlessly removed by biopsy: a forceps is passed through the scope, its jaws are closed around the polyp, and the forceps is pulled back until the polyp is removed (figure 3.4). Larger polyps are re-

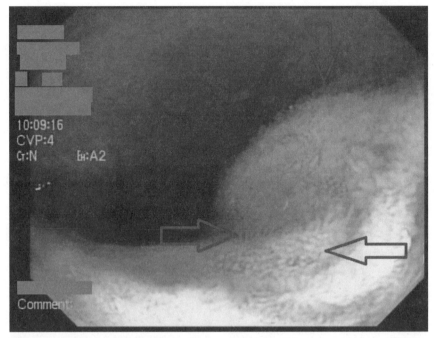

10:09:16
CVP:4
Cr:N   Eh:A2

Comment:

Figure 3.3.   The terminal ileum, the last part of the small intestine. Note that the surface is covered with tiny projections called villi (arrows).
Source: David M. Novick, *Terminal Ileum,* July 2016.

moved by snare and cautery, in which the polyp is lassoed by a wire loop which is then tightened. Then low-level electric current is passed through the wire, allowing the loop to cut the tissue as it is further tightened. Once detached, the polyp is suctioned through the scope and captured in a plastic trap so it can be sent for analysis. This procedure is referred to as polypectomy.

Polypectomy of relatively small polyps can be done with the snare wire but without cautery, a technique with a lower risk of complications (see chapter 6, "Colonoscopy: Risks, Alternatives, and Barriers," for a discussion of complications of colonoscopy).

Some large polyps or tumors are more safely removed surgically. When the physician encounters a large polyp that either cannot be completely removed, or requires surgery, he or she may inject dye at the site. Such tattoos (figure 3.4) allow the site to be easily recognized at a follow-up colonoscopy or subsequent surgery.

Another intervention that can be done during a colonoscopy is the placement of an endoclip. An endoclip is a metal clip with two jaws that are closed over an area of the inner membrane of the colon. The endoclip can pinch off an area that is bleeding, or close up an area that might rupture or perforate. It

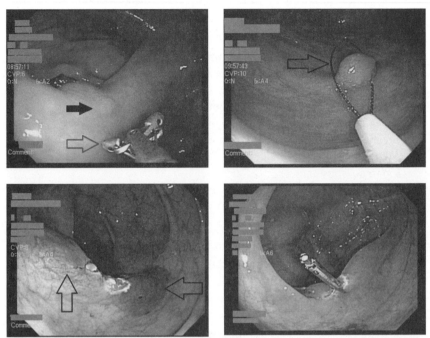

Figure 3.4. Polyp removal, tattooing, and clip placement. Upper left: Forceps (open arrow) being positioned to remove a small polyp (solid arrow). Upper right: Snare wire (arrow) about to be closed around a polyp. Lower left: Ink has been injected (arrows) where a polyp has been removed, allowing the site to be identified at surgery or follow-up colonoscopy. Lower right: An endoclip has been placed to close up a polypectomy site. In the lower images, the areas between the ink spots, or near the base of the clip, represent colon tissue that was cauterized in order to remove a large polyp.
Source: David M. Novick, *Forceps,* July 2016.

is important to know if an endoclip has been placed, because if so, you should not have a magnetic resonance imaging (MRI) procedure for a certain time period thereafter, usually six to eight weeks. Most clips have fallen off and are passed in the stool, and if not, most are MRI safe after that period of time. Check with your gastroenterologist if a clip has been placed.

You should know that, even if you are awake during a biopsy or polypectomy, you will not feel pain. Discomfort during colonoscopy is mostly caused by the air that is instilled into the colon. You will need to pass this air out after the procedure. It is important to remember that this is room air which has no odor, and passing it out is not only socially acceptable within the endoscopy unit, but also medically necessary to relieve crampy discomfort and let the nurse or doctor know that the colon is functioning normally.

In addition to polyps, many other GI conditions can be diagnosed at colonoscopy. A short list of some of the most common are:

- Diverticulosis (chapter 8, "Diverticulosis and Diverticulitis")
- Ulcerative colitis and Crohn's disease (chapter 10, "Inflammatory Bowel Disease")
- Colon cancer (chapter 7, "Overview of Colon Cancer")
- Other types of colitis, including ischemic colitis, resulting from inadequate blood supply to the colon, and microscopic colitis, in which the colon appears normal but biopsies show inflammation
- Lipomas (fatty tumors)
- Abnormal blood vessels

Biopsies (tissue samples) can be taken using the same forceps described above for small polyps.

See chapter 13, "Evaluation of the Esophagus, Stomach, and Small Intestine," for information on cleaning and disinfection of GI endoscopes.

CASE REPORT: AN UNEXPECTED FINDING

Wanda, fifty-one, came in for a colonoscopy for evaluation of blood-on-wiping and constipation alternating with diarrhea. Dr. Fioretti, the gastroenterologist, removed several small polyps from the left colon and did some biopsies for possible colitis. Diverticulosis (chapter 8) and large internal hemorrhoids were seen. When Dr. Fioretti reached the cecum, she saw a most unexpected object.

An earring was resting on the surface of the cecum, unattached in any way (see figure 3.5). Dr. Fioretti and Nurse Lucinda easily grabbed it with a net and carefully withdrew the scope, the net, and the earring. Later, Lucinda carefully washed the earring and could see a bright diamond mounted on it (story continued at end of chapter 4).

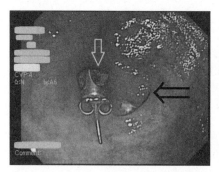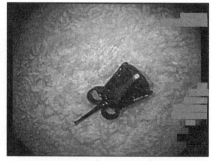

Figure 3.5. A diamond earring found in the cecum. Left image: The earring is resting in the cecum. It was not attached to the tissue of the cecum and was easily removed. Arrow pointing down: Diamond. Arrow pointing left: The appendiceal orifice. Right image: The earring resting on a towel after removal from the patient.

Source: Marios C. Pouagare, *Earring in Cecum*, July 2016. © Archaeopteryx Media LLC.

TAKE-HOME MESSAGES

- A "time out," modeled after airline industry procedures, ensures that the correct procedure is being done on the indicated patient.
- The goal of colonoscopy is to find and remove polyps and to diagnose other GI disorders.
- Small polyps are removed during colonoscopy using biopsy forceps. Large polyps can be removed with a snare wire, usually with cautery. Some very large polyps should be removed surgically.
- Areas of inflammation can be biopsied.
- Emergencies and unexpected events do occur. Gastroenterologists, GI nurses, and other team members are trained to handle them.

4

Recovery after Colonoscopy

After your procedure, you will be wheeled back to the recovery area, where a nurse will monitor you to ensure that you remain stable and recover uneventfully. In recovery, you will be reconnected to monitoring equipment to check your blood pressure, pulse, and oxygen saturation. Although some people are already awake at the end of the procedure, most are still sedated or somewhere between awake and asleep.

Your most important job at this point is to pass air out through the rectum. The nurse will encourage you to do so. If you are at all conscious during this phase, remember that you are only passing room air. In this setting, it is not only socially acceptable but also medically necessary! And, once you pass the air, you will feel much better. Most of the time, due to the lingering effects of the sedation, you will not remember the time when you were advised to pass gas.

Once you have passed some air, the nurse or medical assistant will give you some clear liquid to drink. When you are sufficiently awake, your IV will be removed, and you will get dressed and your doctor will discuss the results of your procedure with you. It is best to have another person with you for this discussion. There is still sedative or anesthetic in the body, which may cause you to forget what is being said. If you have received midazolam (Versed) during your procedure, you are especially likely to have amnesia for the after-procedure discussion. We have had patients that received Versed call the office and complain that no one spoke to them after their procedure, because they did not remember the discussion that took place. When the findings are particularly complex or serious, a follow-up visit in four to seven days after the pathology results are back is appropriate. Many practices and hospitals have a secure online site for each patient, called a portal. After you have signed up for the portal, you will be able to check your results. Please review such results with your doctor, as his or her interpretation may be essential for proper understanding. Remember that a biopsy does not mean cancer. It simply means a tissue sample, the vast majority of which are not cancer.

WHAT CAUSES POLYPS?

This question comes up frequently in conversations after colonoscopy. As in many human diseases, there are multiple factors that contribute to the development of colon polyps. The factors below are thought to increase the odds of developing adenomas, the type of polyp that can progress to colon cancer. These factors can be divided into two broad categories: biological and environmental (see table 4.1). The biological factors are inherited and cannot be changed, with the exception being inflammatory bowel disease (Crohn's disease or ulcerative colitis; see chapter 10, "Crohn's Disease and Ulcerative Colitis: Inflammatory Bowel Disease"), which can be treated if present. The environmental factors can be modified.

Table 4.1.　Factors that promote the development of colon polyps

Biological	Environmental
• Increasing age	• Smoking
• Male	• Alcohol use, especially heavy
• African American	• Overweight/obesity
• Colon cancer or adenomatous polyps in first-degree relatives (parents, siblings, children)	• Sedentary lifestyle
	• Diet high in fat and red meat, low in fiber
• Lynch syndrome or other genetic disorders (see chapter 5, "Putting Colonoscopy in Perspective: The Evidence, Quality Issues, and Surveillance Intervals")	• Diabetes, especially if not well controlled
	• Use of aspirin or nonsteroidal anti-inflammatory medications*
• A personal history of colon cancer or adenomatous polyps	
• Inflammatory bowel disease	

*In contrast to all of the other factors, this one is protective: these medications are associated with reduced numbers of colon polyps. Their use solely for this purpose is not recommended because the effect is small and these medications can cause serious side effects including GI tract bleeding.

Please note that your gastroenterologist may not be available at the moment that you are awake and anxious to go home. He or she may be doing another procedure, and neither your procedure nor the next one should be rushed. Sometimes it's the driver who gets "antsy," but patience at this stage is recommended.

During this time, a nurse or medical assistant will review important safety precautions for the remainder of the day. You will be reminded not to drive, use any equipment that requires alertness, or sign any documents. Don't think that you can get away with driving; our staff has called the police a few times for this. You will also be told that you may eat at home, but not in a restaurant.

People often ask why they can't go out to eat after their procedure. After all, they haven't had solid food for more than twenty-four hours and often are totally obsessed with food. There are two reasons. First, traces of the sedative remain in the body for many hours. If you go to a restaurant, you might get dizzy, hit your head on the hard table, and get carried out by the rescue squad with everyone staring at you. Second, air is placed into the colon by the doctor, in order to enhance visualization. It is normal and desirable to pass this air out afterward, and although it has no odor, it is not silent. If you go to a restaurant, do you really want people looking around to see who let the air out?

CASE REPORT: AN UNEXPECTED FINDING (CONTINUED FROM CHAPTER 3)

After Wanda woke up, Nurse Lucinda, Dr. Fioretti, and Wanda's sister, Ruth, sat down with her in a consultation room. Lucinda said, handing her the earring, "We have a present for you, and we think it is very valuable."

Wanda put her hand over her mouth to stop herself from screaming. "Oh! I can't believe it. I thought it was gone. I've been looking for this earring for months. Oh! I'm so excited!"

Ruth interjected, "Remember how you thought the dog ate it?"

Wanda put her hand to her mouth again, this time hoping she wasn't turning red. "Oh! I was so sure that Duchess ate it! I even went through her poo for weeks. I can't believe it!" Composing herself somewhat, she said to Lucinda and Dr. Fioretti, "These earrings are priceless. My grandmother gave them to me many years ago for graduation."

"So," said Ruth, "where exactly did you find the earring?"

"It was sitting there in the cecum, the end point of the scope's journey through the colon," said Dr. Fioretti.

"I can't thank you enough," said Wanda.

"All's well that ends well," added Lucinda.

CASE REPORT: "I CAN DRIVE. I FEEL FINE."

Pete had a colonoscopy with conscious sedation. After the procedure, his wife, Jenny, was driving him home, and Pete kept saying things like, "I'm OK to drive," "I feel fine," and "These doctors don't know what they are talking about with all their restrictions." Jenny told him to relax and kept driving, but he kept on with his complaints. She finally had to firmly declare, "The doctor said you are not driving, and I say you are not driving, and that's final!" Then, Pete said that he was really thirsty and wanted a cup of coffee. Jenny pulled into a gas station, and Pete quickly dove out of the car to go inside and get the coffee. Jenny was more than a little frustrated with his attitude and decided to stay in the car and read her book. Pete seemed to be in there a long time, but eventually he came out with the coffee. She drove him home and he went to sleep. When he woke up, he didn't remember anything of the procedure or getting the coffee.

A few weeks later, he got his credit card bill and saw a charge for $70 from the gas station on the day of his colonoscopy. He couldn't understand how he could be charged $70 when he only had a cup of coffee. After several calls to the station, he went over there and met with the manager, who had pulled the records and the surveillance video from that time. The clerk on duty remembered seeing Pete in line to get his coffee and getting into a friendly conversation with another customer. He paid for the other guy's gasoline and snacks along with the cup of coffee for himself! Pete told me that he really learned a lesson from this experience, and that he will adhere to doctors' instructions much more carefully in the future.

TAKE-HOME MESSAGES

- After a colonoscopy, it is expected that you will pass air out through the rectum. Don't hold back.
- You may not drive or go to a restaurant after your procedure. Do not schedule anything for the rest of that day or night.
- Have someone that you trust accompany you when the doctor reviews your findings after the procedure, since you may not remember that conversation.
- Biopsy results take a few days, and occasionally longer, to become available. Many practices and hospitals have an online portal through which you can view your results. Be sure to discuss the results with your doctor, as his or her judgment is necessary for proper interpretation.
- Many factors can increase the odds of colon polyps. If you have polyps that are adenomas, and thus potentially precancerous, discuss the steps that you can take with your gastroenterologist and your primary care doctor.

5

Putting Colonoscopy in Perspective

The Evidence, Quality Issues, and Surveillance Intervals

If you are considering colonoscopy but want to know if it is really worth all the fuss and bother, this section is for you. I will summarize the data from five landmark studies which show the benefit of colon cancer screening with colonoscopy. I will also review assessment of quality in colonoscopy, with regard to how likely each doctor's procedures are to achieve the goal of colon cancer prevention. Appropriate intervals for follow-up colonoscopies are also summarized. Before reading any further, please remember that you should make all medical decisions in consultation with your personal physician.

Screening colonoscopy is based on the following concepts:

- Colon cancers arise from a common type of polyp, or growth, in the colon called an **adenoma**.
- Removing adenomas will prevent cancer from developing and will save lives.

The most common types of polyps are adenomas, including villous and sessile serrated adenomas, and hyperplastic polyps. Adenomas, or adenomatous polyps, are **benign (non-cancerous)** growths. Most adenomas do no harm, but a small percentage of them will keep growing and turn into cancer. Villous adenomas tend to be larger and have a greater risk of becoming cancer. Sessile serrated adenomas are a newly described type of polyp, discussed below. The other major type of benign polyps, known as hyperplastic polyps, almost never becomes cancer. However, there is some uncertainty as to whether multiple large hyperplastic polyps lead to increased cancer risk. It is not possible to distinguish adenomatous and hyperplastic polyps by their appearance during colonoscopy, and it is therefore standard practice to remove *all* polyps. Only after the polyp tissue is viewed under a microscope by a pathologist do we know if it was adenomatous or hyperplastic, and benign or malignant.

WHAT IS A SESSILE SERRATED ADENOMA?

Sessile serrated adenomas, also known as sessile serrated polyps, are very flat polyps which are difficult to see, as they may blend in with surrounding normal colon tissue (see figure 3.1 in chapter 3, "The Colonoscopy"). They most commonly occur in the proximal, or right colon, i.e., the last part of the colon reached by the scope. They have potential for malignant change which increases with larger size, and because they are more frequently missed, they may cause many of the cancers that appear after a screening colonoscopy (interval cancers).[1] The management is similar to other adenomas, but this type of polyp has only recently been recognized. Guidelines may change when more studies become available.

The term "serrated" refers to a sawtooth pattern seen under the microscope. A serrated pattern is also seen in hyperplastic polyps, and it is only in the last ten years or so that there has been widespread recognition of sessile serrated adenomas and how they can be distinguished from hyperplastic polyps.

The following five landmark studies show that screening colonoscopy can greatly reduce your risk of colon cancer. Colon cancer is the third leading cause of cancer deaths in the United States, and about 50,000 Americans die from colon cancer annually. That's almost as many deaths **each year** as those Americans who died during the entire Vietnam War. The lifetime risk of colon cancer in the United States is about 5 percent.[2] The death rate for colon cancer in the United States is exceeded only by lung, breast (in women), and prostate cancer (in men).[3] However, no screening test, including colonoscopy, can detect and eliminate 100 percent of adenomatous polyps. Colon cancer cannot be completely prevented, but getting screened for colon cancer will greatly increase your odds of avoiding this serious disease. See chapter 7, "Overview of Colon Cancer," for an overview of what happens when colon cancer is diagnosed.

STATISTICS FOR 2014–2016 FROM
THE AMERICAN CANCER SOCIETY[4,5]

- 136,830 new cases of colon cancer expected in 2014; 134,490 are expected in 2016.
- 50,310 deaths from colon cancer expected in 2014; 49,190 are expected in 2016.
- 60 percent of colon cancer cases and 70 percent of deaths are in persons age sixty-five or older.
- Rates of new cases of, and deaths from, colon cancer are higher in African Americans and lower in Asians and Pacific Islanders.
- 19 percent of new cases of colon cancer in men, and 29 percent in women, are in persons age eighty or older.

There are usually no signs and symptoms in people with colon adenomas, even when these adenomas are large (increasing size of colon polyps correlates with increased risk of malignant change). Colon cancer may have *no symptoms until an advanced stage is reached.* There may be no visible blood, pain, or change in bowel habits, even in cancers that have already spread (usually to lymph nodes or the liver). So, there is no logic in saying "I feel fine" or "I'll wait until I have symptoms" as a reason not to do colonoscopy or another method of colon cancer screening.

The following studies provide evidence that colonoscopy can prevent colon cancer and thereby save lives.

Study #1: Does removing adenomatous polyps by colonoscopy prevent colon cancer?

Before the advent of colon cancer screening of healthy people with no symptoms, the National Polyp Study was initiated to study whether colonoscopic polypectomy (polyp removal) could reduce the incidence of colon cancer. This study, published in 1993 as part of the National Polyp Study, included 1,418 patients who had a colonoscopy showing one or more adenomas, but not cancer.[6] These were average-risk patients with no family history of colon cancer. They were followed for an average of 5.9 years, and their incidence of colon cancer was determined and compared with three reference groups. The first reference group had polyps identified on barium enema between 1965 and 1970, but not removed. The second group had rectal adenomas removed from 1957 to 1980, when colonoscopy was not widely available. The third group consisted of average-risk people in the general population who participated in a National Cancer Institute survey that took place at the same time as this study.

Since the study included 1,418 patients, it was predicted that cancer would develop in 48.3 patients based on the first reference group, 43.4 patients based on the second group, and 20.7 patients based on the third group. In actuality, there were **only five** cancers found on follow-up colonoscopy: three at three years after the initial colonoscopy, one at six years, and one at seven years. Based on those three reference groups, the authors calculated that the **incidence of colon cancer was reduced by 90 percent, 88 percent, and 76 percent, respectively**. These data show that colonoscopy with removal of adenomas significantly reduces the incidence of colon cancer.

Study #2: Does removing adenomatous polyps by colonoscopy save lives?

This question was addressed in a 2012 report from the National Polyp Study.[7] The investigators studied all patients in their database who had a polypectomy between 1980 and 1990. There were 2,602 patients with an adenoma and 773 patients with non-adenomatous polyps. They compared the death rate from colon cancer in these two groups with a reference group of the general population. During a median of 15.8 years of follow-up, there were **twelve** deaths from colon cancer in the patients who had adenomas removed at colonoscopy, compared with **twenty-five** deaths expected in the general population. Also, in the first ten years of the study, the colon cancer death rate was similar to that in patients whose polyps were not adenomas (a low-risk group in whom few cancers would be expected). This study shows that death from colon cancer can be prevented by removal of adenomas.

Studies #3–4: Has the increased use of colon cancer screening in the last decade had any effect on the incidence of colon cancer in the general population?

The American Cancer Society provides the following data from 2001 to 2010:[8]

- Overall **colon cancer incidence declined** by an average rate of 3.4 percent per year.
- In adults age fifty or over, **colon cancer incidence declined** by 3.9 percent annually (total decrease for the decade was 30 percent).
- In adults age sixty-five or older, **colon cancer incidence declined** by 3.6 percent annually from 2001 to 2008 and 7.2 percent from 2008 to 2010.
- In adults age fifty to seventy-five, **screening colonoscopy increased** from 19 percent to 55 percent from 2000 to 2010.

- **Colon cancer death rate declined** by 3 percent per year in 2001–2010.
- Colon cancer incidence increased by 1.1 percent per year in persons **under** age fifty, a group thought to be at very low risk for colon cancer.

In another study, a group of investigators studied the incidence of colon cancer over three decades (1976–2009), along with rates of colon cancer screening.[9] They found that screening, by all methods, including colonoscopy, increased from 34.8 percent to 66.1 percent during 1987–2010 (the years for which screening data were available). They estimate that **because of screening**, the incidence of colon cancer decreased such that **550,000 cases were prevented** in the three decades they studied. Although the decrease in incidence was for cancers in both early and late stages, the greatest decline was for late-stage disease (cancer which has spread to lymph nodes or distant organs such as the liver). Also, the decline in distal or left-sided colon cancers, those most frequently detected by screening (see the "Quality Issues" section later in this chapter), was much greater than that for proximal or right-sided cancers. The authors believe that these data strongly support the idea that **colon cancer screening is the major factor contributing to the decrease in colon cancer incidence**. Other factors, including dietary changes, less cigarette smoking, and widespread use of aspirin and other non-steroidal anti-inflammatory medications, may also contribute to the decreasing incidence of colon cancer.[10]

Colonoscopies are classified as diagnostic or screening based on whether a person is or is not having symptoms. Cancer can be found in both cases. If a cancer is found, the patient should be referred for surgery with the intent to cure (see chapter 7). Even if it is known that the cancer has spread to other tissues and is no longer curable, surgery is often recommended to prevent the possibility of a bowel obstruction. **Diagnosis of curable cancers is another benefit of colonoscopy,** above and beyond the prevention information discussed previously. The following study compares patients who had their cancer diagnosed by screening versus those who had it diagnosed because of symptoms.

Study #5: Does screening colonoscopy detect cancers at an earlier stage than colonoscopy done for symptoms?

Researchers looked at all patients who had colon cancer surgery at a large hospital.[11] The study covered an eight-year period ending in 2011 and included 1,071 patients, including 217 who had their cancer diagnosed by screening colonoscopy. The others did not undergo screening and either waited until they had symptoms or had other reasons to get a colonoscopy.

The patients who had screening colonoscopy had less invasive cancers, less spread to lymph nodes, less spread to organs outside the intestines, lower death rates, and longer survival. At any given stage of cancer, the survival rate was better in the screening group. The investigators conclude that, in addition to preventing colon cancer by removing adenomas, screening colonoscopy detects cancers at lower stages and leads to better survival in patients with colon cancer, when compared with colonoscopy done for symptoms or other reasons.

Quality Issues

While no research study is perfect, these results show that colon cancer screening can significantly reduce the incidence and death rate of colon cancer. Now that the importance of screening colonoscopy has been established, the next step is to maximize the benefits of the procedure by ensuring quality. Several recent studies have shown that the benefit of colonoscopy is greater in the distal colon (the first part examined when the scope is inserted; the left colon) than the proximal colon (the last part of the colon reached by the scope; the right colon).[12] This discrepancy is mainly a result of quality factors, which can be improved, and to a lesser extent biologic factors, such as more aggressive progression of proximal polyps to cancer. Quality factors are mainly under the control of the endoscopist, and across the United States programs are measuring these factors and providing feedback to doctors so they can further improve.

As a patient, it is important for you to know that quality factors for colonoscopy are:[13]

- Reaching the cecum (denotes a complete exam)
- Taking enough time to remove all polyps, especially proximal colon polyps, which may be flatter and harder to see (see previous section on sessile serrated adenomas and figure 3.1 in chapter 3)
- Complete removal of polyps
- An excellent bowel prep, which makes all of colon visible

Quality can be measured by the adenoma detection rate (ADR) and cecal intubation rate (rate of reaching the cecum, the last part of the colon that the colonoscope reaches), and these rates will soon, if not already, be available to consumers. The ADR is the percentage of colonoscopies done by a doctor or group that detect one or more adenomas. The standard for the ADR in 2015 is 20 percent or higher in women and 30 percent or higher in men. Much higher rates are possible. In a recent study, the top 20 percent of gastroenterologists had an average ADR of 39 percent for all patients.[14] The study showed a strong correlation between a high ADR and a low incidence of subsequent colon cancers (both proximal and distal), advanced colon cancers (evidence of spread to lymph nodes or distant organs), and colon cancer deaths.

IMPORTANT QUESTIONS

- Does your gastroenterologist measure his or her ADR?
- Is the ADR posted on the practice website?
- Does the practice use a registry to measure ADR and other important indices, such as cecal intubation rate? A registry collects data from many physicians in a standard way and calculates quality measures.

Table 5.1. Dr. David M. Novick's Adenoma Detection Rate from the GIQuIC Registry*

Year	Male	Female	Total
2014**	60.0%	48.4%	54.6%
2015	50.4%	35.3%	42.8%
2016***	56.2%	48.8%	52.1%
Benchmark	30%	20%	25%

*Includes all patients age fifty and over having screening colonoscopy. Pronounced "GI Quick," this registry is a joint project of the American College of Gastroenterology and the American Society of Gastrointestinal Endoscopy.
**Last nine months.
***First five months.

WARNING: Beware of insurance company-sponsored "quality" assessments. These may appear on websites for insurance plan members. They may be cost-containment measures masquerading as quality measures. In other words, what they consider as quality may be the cheapest but not the best. Are the criteria clearly stated? See if they include ADR and cecal intubation rate.

When Should Colon Cancer Screening Be Done?

The first colonoscopy should be done at the following times:

- Average-risk adults: age fifty.
- Family history of colon cancer: age forty, or ten years earlier than the age of the family member with the cancer. For example, if a man had colon

cancer at age forty-two, his children should start colon cancer screening at age thirty-two.
- Family history of adenomatous polyps: same as for family history of colon cancer. Note: people often report a family history of polyps, but very few report a family history of adenomas. If you have polyps, it will be most helpful to your family if you find out the type of polyp and share this information with them.
- African American men or women: age forty-five. The risk of colon cancer is higher.[15]

For colon cancer screening, the relevant family history is in **first-degree relatives**: parents, siblings, and children. Having another affected relative such as an aunt, uncle, cousin, or grandparent does not increase your risk, but having several of them may do so. There are several familial syndromes in which multiple family members in one or more generations have colon cancer. More rigorous screening protocols are needed for these, the most common of which is Lynch syndrome.

LYNCH SYNDROME[16]

- Affected individuals have mutations in certain genes called mismatch repair genes.
- The lifetime risk for colon cancer is 30–74 percent for some mutations, and 10–22 percent for others.
- Colon cancer occurs at much younger ages in Lynch syndrome patients.
- The progression from adenoma to cancer is much more rapid in Lynch syndrome compared with non-familial colon cancer.
- Lynch syndrome patients are also at risk for certain cancers other than in the colon. Endometrial (uterine) cancer is the most common. Others are stomach, ovary, pancreas, ureter, kidney, biliary tract, and small intestine.
- Lynch syndrome should be considered in anyone with a personal or family history (first-degree relative) of any of the above cancers before age fifty, colon polyps (adenomas) before age fifty, or three or more relatives (including cousins, aunts, uncles, and grandparents) who had colon cancer.
- The diagnosis of Lynch syndrome can be made by testing tumor tissue for mutations, blood tests, and genetic counseling. In 2014, several of the GI societies recommended that colon cancer tissue be tested for Lynch syndrome mutations in all patients with colon cancer.
- Patients (or first-degree relatives of patients) with Lynch syndrome need aggressive screening for colon, endometrial, ovarian, gastric, and urinary tract cancer.

Surveillance

These recommendations, and those that follow, are based on published medical guidelines and may not apply to every individual.[17-19] The judgment of the physician, based on the specific needs and circumstances of the patient, takes precedence.

The risk of an adenoma becoming malignant depends on the size of the polyp and certain features seen under the microscope. Advanced, or high-risk, adenomas are those that are 10 millimeters in diameter or larger, or have villous features or high-grade dysplasia (see glossary for details) on pathologic evaluation.[20]

The timing of follow-up (surveillance) colonoscopies depends on the results of the initial colonoscopy and the family history. Most patients will fall into one of the following categories for their second colonoscopy:

- **Ten years**: No adenomatous polyps or cancer on the initial colonoscopy *and* no family history of colon cancer or adenomatous polyps.
- **Five years**: One or two small (less than 1 centimeter) adenomatous polyps and/or a family history of colon cancer or adenomatous polyps.
- **Three years**: One or more large (1 centimeter or larger) adenomatous polyps, three or more adenomas of any size, or adenomas with high-risk features (villous pathology or high-grade dysplasia).
- **Less than three years**: More than ten adenomas.

CAN YOU GO FROM HIGH RISK TO LOW RISK?

Yes. If on your first colonoscopy you had one or two small adenomas and have no polyps on your second colonoscopy, you are now average risk. Your next screening colonoscopy is recommended in ten years.[21]

Colon cancer screening is continued until at least age seventy-five. Thereafter it is not routine, but depends on the health of the patient, the results of previous colonoscopies, and the informed decision of the patient. It is rarely done after age eighty-five, but many people aged seventy-five to eighty-five are in excellent health and have a life expectancy of more than ten years. Colonoscopy in such individuals is reasonable and may prevent many of the cancers that appear in the eighth, ninth, and tenth decades of life. Complications of colonoscopy are also more common in the elderly. A recent study suggests that average-risk individuals who have had *no prior colon cancer screening* will benefit from colon cancer screening up to age eighty-six; if they have no significant medical conditions, colonoscopy was found to be beneficial up to age eighty-three; and less invasive tests (fecal occult blood testing or sigmoidoscopy, see chapter 6, "Colonoscopy: Risks, Alternatives, and Barriers) to age eighty-six.[22] Articles in the popular press saying that colonoscopy is "an unnecessary test" for anyone over seventy-five do the elderly a great disservice.

All of these recommendations are based on the assumption that the colonoscopy is done with an excellent bowel prep and high-quality observation. After a poor prep, colonoscopy should be repeated within one year at the latest.

CASE REPORT: IF YOU BET REAL MONEY, YOU'VE GOT TO FOLLOW THROUGH

"One of my patients, whom I'll call Kenny, had a cancer in the cecum, about two years ago," said Dr. Fioretti. "He had surgery, and all of his lymph nodes were negative. He's been doing fine and had a negative follow-up screening colonoscopy. Every summer, Kenny and three other guys, all over fifty, go see games at baseball stadiums that they have not previously visited. It turned out that none of the other guys had had a colonoscopy. So, two years ago, Kenny told them about his cancer and tried to get them to get screened. When they met again last summer, none of them had done anything, so he bet them each $100 that they wouldn't get a colonoscopy done by this summer. In other words, if they did the colonoscopy they would each get $100. Kenny proposed the bet after they had all had a few beers, and he told me that he was surprised that they all agreed. When they met again the following summer, they all had done the colonoscopy, and he thought he would have to shell out $300. But the interesting thing is that one had a cancer and the other two each had large polyps, and none of them would take the money!"

TAKE-HOME MESSAGES

- Colon cancer may have no symptoms until it has become very large or spread to distant organs. **Do not wait to be tested until you have symptoms; it may be too late.**
- Colon cancers begin as benign polyps called adenomas.
- Removing adenomas by colonoscopy results in significantly fewer colon cancers and a reduced rate of death from colon cancer.
- People who have their cancers discovered by screening colonoscopy have less advanced disease, a lower death rate, and longer survival

than those who have their cancer discovered after colonoscopy done for symptoms.

- African Americans should commence colon cancer screening at age forty-five. Greater efforts in publicizing this are needed.
- It is not true that colonoscopy after age seventy-five is an "unnecessary test." The guidelines say that the decision should be based on the individual needs of the patient. For someone over seventy-five who has never had colon cancer screening and is in good health, colonoscopy should be done, at least through the early eighties.
- The adenoma detection rate accurately reflects the quality of colonoscopy that an individual doctor provides.

6

Colonoscopy

Risks, Alternatives, and Barriers

The first five chapters have described and advocated for colonoscopy as the most effective means to reduce the risk of colon cancer. Colonoscopy is an invasive procedure, in that an instrument is placed inside the body. Invasive procedures have risks, discussed here, that need to be understood in order to make an informed decision. These risks are one of the many reasons that some have sought alternatives to colonoscopy, and the available alternatives are also reviewed here. Other reasons why people avoid having colonoscopy are discussed in the section below, "Barriers to Colonoscopy."

RISKS OF COLONOSCOPY

Colonoscopy is generally considered to be a safe procedure, and complications are rare. The most serious risk of colonoscopy is perforation, or puncture of the colon, which is suspected when a patient experiences significant abdominal pain and extreme bloating, and is unable to pass air after the procedure. These symptoms may be evident immediately after the procedure or later, usually within one to three days. If a patient in an endoscopy center is suspected of having had a perforation, he or she should be sent immediately to a hospital. Emergency surgery is usually needed, although in recent years, some perforations have been closed non-surgically with endoclips. Perforation can lead to infection, as residual stool in the colon can then enter the abdominal cavity. Because the colon has been mostly cleaned out by the bowel prep, these infections can usually be successfully treated with antibiotics. Carefully selected patients with colon perforation following colonoscopy can be treated without surgery using antibiotics and bowel rest (nothing by mouth).

Bleeding may occur after colonoscopy, usually after removal of a large polyp. A subsequent colonoscopy will identify the site, and the bleeding can be controlled by injecting drugs that constrict blood vessels. A heater probe to cauterize the bleeding vessel may be used, and/or placing of a clip. Aspiration of stomach contents, i.e., the inhalation of stomach contents that have traveled up from the esophagus into the throat, is a rare complication of colonoscopy that can cause serious pneumonia. Aspiration pneumonia is more common, though still very rare, with endoscopy of the upper GI tract (see chapter 13, "Evaluation of the Esophagus, Stomach, and Small Intestine"). Other reported complications are fever and abdominal pain due to multiple polypectomies (post-polypectomy syndrome) and cardiopulmonary complications, including breathing difficulty, aspiration, abnormal heart rhythm, and heart attack. Rupture of the spleen is a very rare complication. Table 6.1 shows the published rates of colonoscopy complications.

Table 6.1.   Rates of Complications of Colonoscopy[1]

Complication	Rate
Perforation—all colonoscopies	0.1–0.3%*
Perforation—screening colonoscopies	0.01%
Bleeding	0.1–0.6%**
Cardiopulmonary	0.9%
Post-polypectomy syndrome	0.003–0.1%
Death—all causes***	0.07%
Death—specifically related to colonoscopy***	0.007%

*0.1% is one in 1,000.
**Risk increases with removal of polyps, especially large polyps.
***Within 30 days of the colonoscopy.

ALTERNATIVES TO COLONOSCOPY
FOR COLON CANCER SCREENING

You get that colon cancer screening is important, but you just can't bring yourself to allow a five-foot-long scope to be inserted into your rectum, even though you won't remember it because of the anesthesia. Are there alternatives? The answer is a qualified "yes," with the caveat that any alternative colon cancer screening method will mandate a colonoscopy in the event of abnormal results. So consider the following options, but be aware that you may wind up scheduling a colonoscopy anyway. Many people favor colonoscopy because it's "one-stop shopping." You are evaluated and treated with (and charged for) one procedure. The main alternatives include the following:

Flexible Sigmoidoscopy

Flexible sigmoidoscopy is the use of a short scope that evaluates at most one-third of the colon, the distal (left) portion. It is safer than a colonoscopy and less expensive, as it can be done in an office with no sedation. For screening purposes, it is done every five years, and it can be combined with stool testing. The lack of sedation will be unacceptable to many people. Flexible sigmoidoscopy will prevent most distal colon cancers. It may also prevent some proximal (right colon) cancers, assuming that a full colonoscopy is done when adenomas are detected in the left colon by the sigmoidoscopy. Despite the limitations of colonoscopy in the proximal colon discussed previously, high-quality colonoscopy will detect more proximal adenomas and cancers than any other method.

Stool Tests

The newer stool tests, known collectively as fecal immunochemical testing (FIT), detect amounts of blood in the stool that are too small to be visible. In contrast to earlier occult blood tests, FIT tests are not affected by taking low-dose aspirin. As a screening test, FIT is done once per year. FIT will detect most cancers and some advanced adenomas. A positive test warrants a colonoscopy.

Stool DNA tests measure human tumor DNA that falls off of the tumor during its growth. Some versions of this test are still in development, but promise greater accuracy, especially in detecting advanced adenomas. They are more expensive than FIT. The first stool DNA test, Cologuard, was approved for colon cancer screening of average-risk people in August 2014. If the stool DNA test is negative, colonoscopy is avoided and the stool test is repeated in three years, but you lose the preventive benefit of removing adenomas. Further advances in this technology are likely in the future.

Virtual Colonoscopy

Virtual Colonoscopy, also known as CT colonography (CTC), is a computed tomographic (CT) scan (see glossary) of the colon. It requires not only a bowel prep, but also ingestion of oral contrast which coats the colon. Just before the scan, a probe is inserted into the rectum and carbon dioxide (CO_2) gas is instilled to inflate the colon. The patient lies on the table and moves through the scanner, and images of the colon are obtained. No sedation is required, so it is permissible to drive to and from the procedure. Some patients have minor discomfort from the CO_2 gas, which is used because it dissipates more quickly than room air. An important consideration is radiation exposure, which may be significant when added to previous radiation exposure from CT and other scans that are done frequently these days. A five-year interval is recommended for CTC as a screening modality.

CTC can detect most large (1-centimeter or larger) polyps and cancers, but its accuracy decreases for 6- to 9-millimeter polyps and flat polyps. Polyps 5 millimeters or smaller are not detected with current technology. If a polyp or mass is found on CTC, then colonoscopy will be needed. There is a minimal risk of perforation with CTC. CTC also provides images of the liver, spleen, pancreas, kidneys, and other abdominal organs, which can detect serious pathology but may lead to unnecessary testing for more minor abnormalities.

Because of these concerns, CTC has not been approved as a screening test. It will usually be covered by insurance only in the event that colonoscopy was attempted but was incomplete. Otherwise, it is available on a cash-only basis. CTC is attractive to many consumers because of the low risk, lack of sedation, and accuracy for cancers and large polyps. Greater use of CTC would increase the overall screening rate. It is likely that improvements in technology will eventually render CTC acceptable for colon cancer screening.

Capsule Endoscopy of the Colon

In early 2014, capsule endoscopy was approved for visualization of the colon for patients whose colonoscopy was not successful in reaching the cecum (incomplete colonoscopy). It has not been approved as a primary screening method. It is performed similarly to small bowel capsule endoscopy, as described in chapter 13. It has many of the advantages of virtual colonoscopy—non-invasive, done without sedation—and, in addition, has no radiation exposure. The main limitation is that it will not visualize as completely as the standard or virtual colonoscopy. If polyps are found by this method, a decision must be made to proceed with another attempt at colonoscopy, a surgical consultation, or a repeat capsule endoscopy of the colon after an observation period.

BARRIERS TO COLONOSCOPY

This section addresses the many reasons that people give for not having a colonoscopy. **These are all legitimate concerns that should be discussed**

with your gastroenterologist before your procedure. The reasons fall into one of six categories:

- Fear of discomfort
- Fear of embarrassment
- Fear of danger
- Fear of the unknown
- Lifestyle issues
- Fear that screening won't work

Let's start with **fear of discomfort**. There are two major issues: nausea and pain. Nausea is a common problem with the bowel prep. Some people just cannot drink a large volume of fluid. Nausea is less likely with the smaller-volume preps. While the small-volume preps are more expensive than others (see chapter 1, "Preparing for Colonoscopy"), some people feel they are worth every cent. The PEG solution prep (MiraLAX, GlycoLax, among others) can be mixed with most clear liquids, including water. Some people find that the PEG solution doesn't impart a taste, while others disagree. It can change the consistency and may make the drink seem grainy or sandy. If nausea occurs, it is often alleviated by stopping the prep for thirty minutes to an hour before resuming it. Sometimes it may be necessary to switch to another prep. You should call the doctor on call if you absolutely cannot tolerate the prep, or if you are not responding to the prep. **Keep the importance of the prep in mind; a really good one will allow your gastroenterologist to see that difficult-to-spot polyp just before it hides under a fold. Removing it could add years to your life**.

Pain is another concern. Sedation for colonoscopy is discussed in chapter 2, "Sedation and Anesthesia." It is very effective in almost all people, but there is a small possibility you may experience pain or discomfort and remember it afterward. Your gastroenterologist and anesthesiologist, or nurse anesthetist, are committed to keeping you comfortable, but safety is always the top priority. There may be medical reasons why your sedation is maintained at a lighter level than you might wish it to be, such as changes in oxygen level or blood pressure. Pain after a procedure may tell the doctor something that he or she needs to know, and you should not be reluctant to report it.

Fear of embarrassment may take many forms. For example, fear of the prep causing uncontrolled diarrhea, even though transient, is a problem for some. This aspect of colonoscopy is uncomfortable as well as embarrassing. Sometimes it is best to stay in the bathroom and drink the solution there. Preparing for this possibility by having reading material, music, or a smartphone at hand may help. The diarrhea will not last forever, and at least you know the prep is working!

Another issue is lack of privacy during the procedure. You are exposing parts of your body that are not shown to strangers. I hope that you will be confident in the professionalism of your gastroenterologist and his or her staff. If your privacy concerns would be alleviated by selecting a doctor of the same sex, doing so is reasonable: the important thing is to get your colonoscopy done. If you feel uncomfortable with the doctor to whom you have been referred, you should seriously consider switching doctors or groups—it is your right to do so. It may help to keep in mind that millions of adults have colonoscopies every year. This thought also applies to the concern expressed by some that "I just do not want anything up there." If such feelings are intense, or if there is a history of abuse, then it may be best to use another method of colon cancer screening.

Fear of danger relates to the fact that although complications of colonoscopy are very rare, they do occur. It may be interesting to ask your doctor if he or she has ever had complications when performing the procedure or afterward. If they say never, consider another option or another physician. In reality, the only way a doctor can avoid having any complications at all is to avoid doing procedures. I think people are more reassured by a statement along the lines of "complications are very rare, and we do everything we can to prevent them, but if they do occur we are prepared to manage them in the best possible way."

Whereas it is not uncommon for a patient to say, "I want to be put out," a smaller number will request that sedation be on the lighter side. Some people are terrified of being deeply sedated. The underlying concern may be the lack of control. In this situation, conscious sedation may be preferable to IV anesthesia with propofol. A discussion with the professional who will administer the sedation may go far to alleviate such concerns.

Fear of the unknown: Sometimes health care personnel can forget that, for you, the first colonoscopy is a unique event. It helps if you know what to expect, and providing that knowledge is a major goal of this book. Most people are willing to have a follow-up colonoscopy if the initial one went well. If you have concerns about your previous colonoscopy, please discuss them with your gastroenterologist. It is very likely that accommodations can be made.

Another fear in this category is that something bad may be found, especially cancer. In this case, try to have your intellect rule over your emotions, and not the reverse. Finding cancer sooner can lead to a cure. As discussed in chapter 5, "Putting Colonoscopy in Perspective: The Evidence, Quality Issues, and Surveillance Intervals," Study #5, screening colonoscopy is associated with finding significantly more curable cancers than colonoscopy for symptoms or other reasons. There is a longer survival at every stage of colon cancer when the cancer is diagnosed by screening.

Lifestyle issues may be the most significant barrier to colon cancer screening, and particularly colonoscopy. Everyone is too busy. It is necessary to make time for colonoscopy and the prep. Some gastroenterologists may have weekend hours. Working people may be reluctant to take time off for something that they don't really want to do anyway. There may be financial losses with missing work, especially for those that are hired as independent contractors. If your work has a slower season, you may be more able to do the testing then. There are direct costs of the procedure as well, and there may be additional charges for anesthesia and pathology services. If you have a high-deductible insurance plan, you may incur significant out-of-pocket expenses. Many people have their procedures late in the year when they have partially or completely met their deductible. Your gastroenterologist's office staff should be able to inform you of the expected costs before your procedure. It is often possible to set up payment plans. It is wise to discuss your financial concerns ahead of time.

The Affordable Care Act mandates insurance coverage of colon cancer screening. Screening colonoscopy should be 100 percent covered if done within the established guidelines. However, some insurance companies get around this by recategorizing the procedure as "diagnostic" rather than "screening" if a polyp is found and removed. Deductibles, co-pays, and other charges then apply if the procedure is considered diagnostic. The GI societies are fighting this practice but, as of this writing, it still occurs. If you have symptoms such as bleeding, diarrhea, abdominal pain, etc., your procedure will be considered diagnostic and the above charges will apply. These practices vary among insurance plans and you should consult with them before your colonoscopy, if questions arise.

As previously discussed in chapter 1, you may not drive after a procedure. Finding a driver is a barrier for some. The driver need not stay at the endoscopy facility the entire time that you are there. At minimum, they must drop you off, pick you up, and escort you into your home. It is preferable that they remain with you until you are comfortably situated. As discussed in chapter 4, "Recovery after Colonoscopy," it is best to have another person present for the post-procedure discussion. You are likely to have some residual sedative effects at that point. Of course, this must be someone with whom you are comfortable hearing your personal results. Difficulties can occur in finding a driver, especially one that you trust. A small number of people cannot recruit anyone to help them. Although taking a taxi is not acceptable (chapter 1), there may be specialized transportation services in your community that meet the minimum criteria.

Fear that screening won't work: A final barrier to colon cancer screening is that you may become aware that screening programs for some other cancers have modest or no effectiveness in preventing cancer deaths. A discussion of these controversies is beyond the scope of this book, but they have no relevance to the data on colon cancer screening. Some of the top studies are reviewed in chapter 5 so that you can make an informed decision. There is a strong consensus in the medical community in favor of colon cancer screening, including colonoscopy. The research demonstrates that colon cancer screening saves lives.

CASE REPORT: COLONIC BLEEDING

Samantha, twenty-five, came in for a colonoscopy to evaluate of diarrhea, bleeding, anemia, and weight loss. Her colonoscopy started out routinely, but Dr. Sengupta soon encountered patchy areas of intense inflammation with a granular appearance. There was a particularly severe area of involvement at the splenic flexure, where the colon makes a sharp turn in the left upper quadrant of the abdomen, near the spleen. Dr. Sengupta took a biopsy of this area using a forceps. Suddenly, torrential bleeding occurred. The blood was bright red, and pulsations were seen, suggesting arterial bleeding. Samantha's heart rate increased in response to the active bleeding. In such situations, an endoscopist would try to suction the blood away, visualize the exact site of the bleeding, and inject epinephrine (a medication which constricts blood vessels) at the bleeding site with a very thin needle. In this case, the blood came out so fast that no matter how much Dr. Sengupta suctioned, more blood came so quickly that it was impossible to see the bleeding site for even a fraction of a second. Samantha's heart rate kept increasing. Dr. Sengupta was thinking that he would have to call the emergency squad and send Samantha to the hospital when Becky, the GI nurse, said, "How about spraying the epinephrine?"

"I've heard of that, but would it work with such massive bleeding?" said Dr. Sengupta.

Becky explained that she had seen a few cases of minor bleeding which persisted. The physician had sprayed the epinephrine into the blood, rather than injecting it, and the bleeding stopped. As Dr. Sengupta watched the blood continue to pool, he accepted her suggestion.

Becky quickly got the injection needle and the medication ready. Like using a garden hose, he sprayed the epinephrine into the large, swirling pool of blood. Immediately, the bleeding stopped! He suctioned out the remaining blood, and no bleeding was seen from the biopsy site. He then injected some epinephrine there as a precaution.

"I cannot believe what I have just seen!" he said. Becky just smiled. Dr. Sengupta recalled his mentor in medical school who always told him to listen to the advice of good nurses.

Dr. Sengupta continued the colonoscopy and performed several additional biopsies of intermittently inflamed areas with no problem. He suspected that Samantha had Crohn's disease and thought about how best to explain this to her later.

TAKE-HOME MESSAGES

- There are rare, but definite, risks to colonoscopy. Perforation, bleeding, and cardiopulmonary complications are the most serious. These should be discussed with your doctor.
- There are alternatives to colonoscopy. A specialized CT scan of the colon (virtual colonoscopy) can detect most cancers and some larger polyps.
- Stool DNA tests are more accurate, but more expensive, than tests for blood in the stool. One such test has been approved for screening.
- Ask about small-volume bowel preps, but remember the importance of a good prep, whatever method you use.
- You should trust that your doctor and his or her staff respect your privacy and act in a professional manner. If not, make a change.
- Review your insurance coverage before your procedure.
- Colon cancer screening is very effective and saves lives, regardless of the data for screening for other cancers.
- Complications of colonoscopy, or any GI procedure, may occur. Your gastroenterology team—doctors, nurses, techs, and others—are trained to work together and handle them.

7

Overview of Colon Cancer

If you are diagnosed with colon cancer, it is best to take an optimistic attitude. Remember that many colon cancers can be cured surgically, and proper treatment can improve the odds of survival for most stages of colon cancer. Medical advances continue to occur. There is evidence that a positive mental approach can lead to a better physical outcome. This chapter provides basic information on cancer, background information on the signs and symptoms of colon cancer, the treatment options, and the outlook at various stages of colon cancer.

BASIC FACTS ABOUT CANCER

Cancer is not a single disease but a collection of related diseases. There will be different treatments for various cancers based on the specific biologic features of each one. A common feature of cancer is cells growing and dividing excessively. There are differences between cancer cells and normal cells, one of which is that cancer cells ignore signals to stop dividing.[1]

DNA, or deoxyribonucleic acid, is the chemical that contains hereditary information in humans and most other living things. It contains four nitrogen bases that keep repeating, and the order of these bases makes genes, the units of heredity. Genes provide instructions for your cells to make proteins, leading in turn to many other functions. Some genes control how cells grow (or stop growing), divide, and function, while others correct errors in the DNA that occur when cells divide. Cancer is caused by abnormalities in these genes.[2] Cancer could be considered a disease of damaged DNA.

The cells of the body expend a considerable effort to maintain the DNA and fix any errors that occur over time. Many cancers occur when the genes which code for these repair processes, DNA repair genes, are damaged, and the cell can no longer fix the DNA when errors occur. Lynch syndrome, a form of hereditary colon and other cancers (see chapter 5, "Putting Colonoscopy in Perspective: The Evidence, Quality Issues, and Surveillance Intervals"), occurs when there are abnormalities in the DNA repair genes.

Cancer can cause problems by growing and expanding at the site of origin (primary site), or it can spread, or metastasize, to other parts of the body. If a cancer is localized to a primary site, surgery or radiation therapy are the main treatment options. If the cancer has metastasized, chemotherapy or targeted therapy are commonly used because they can travel through the blood and kill or inhibit cancer cells in multiple locations.

Chemotherapy kills dividing cells. Many side effects of chemotherapy occur because it attacks normal dividing cells as well as cancer cells. Targeted therapy attacks the particular changes in cancer cells that cause them to divide out of control. It works on specific molecules that are associated with the growth, progression, and spread of cancer. Agents of targeted therapy may block cancer cell growth, help the immune system destroy cancer cells, or interfere with a process that the cancer cell needs, all without direct toxicity to the cancer cell or surrounding normal cells.[3,4] Chemotherapy and targeted therapy may be combined. It is hoped that targeted therapy will replace chemotherapy as the predominant type of medication used in cancer treatment.

Cancer screening such as colonoscopy is done to identify cancer at an early stage or precancerous abnormalities such as adenomas. Such early detection will allow for more successful treatment with local therapy, e.g., surgery, and avoid the need for more toxic treatment like chemotherapy.

SIGNS AND SYMPTOMS OF COLON CANCER

Chapter 5 stressed that a person can develop colon cancer and have no symptoms. Some patients with colon cancer, however, are diagnosed because of signs or symptoms. The most common include the following:

- Blood in the stool
- Black stool (melena)
- Abdominal pain
- Change in bowel habits
- Iron deficiency anemia
- Weight loss

- Constipation
- Tenesmus (painful straining at stool) for rectal cancer

Other patients may have a bowel obstruction as the initial symptom because the cancer has blocked the lumen (opening) of the bowel. Those patients will commonly have nausea, vomiting, abdominal pain, or distention. Less commonly, a patient may have metastases (tumor deposits in organs not in direct contact with the colon) at the initial medical evaluation. Colon cancer most commonly metastasizes (spreads) to lymph nodes close to the colon and then to the liver, but it may spread to the lungs, brain, or other sites via the bloodstream or lymphatic channels.

IRON DEFICIENCY ANEMIA—IT'S NOT TIRED BLOOD

Iron deficiency anemia is a decrease in the number and size of red blood cells due to abnormally low levels of iron in the body. It deserves careful medical attention. In all men and in women who have reached menopause, iron deficiency means internal bleeding until proven otherwise. The bleeding is usually in the GI tract. The finding of iron deficiency anemia often leads to the diagnosis of colon cancer or other GI disorders. Iron deficiency anemia can be normal in a woman who is having menstrual periods, but not necessarily.

EVALUATION, STAGING, AND TREATMENT OF COLON CANCER

Most cases of colon cancer are diagnosed or confirmed by colonoscopy and biopsy of a mass in the colon. What happens next? A CT scan of the abdomen is recommended to determine whether the cancer has spread to lymph nodes or the liver, and a blood test of liver enzymes may be obtained as an indirect measure of liver involvement. Another test that is often performed at this point is the carcinoembryonic antigen, or CEA.[5] CEA is a protein produced in a developing fetus and in certain cancers, most prominently in colon cancer. In patients with colon cancer, CEA correlates with the amount of cancer in the body. It is often referred to as a "tumor marker," a term that can be misleading since CEA cannot reliably diagnose colon cancer—its value is in detecting recurrent colon cancer after surgery. The test is done before surgery as a baseline. Levels of CEA after surgery or during chemotherapy may correlate with prognosis and the response to the treatment. People with colon cancer and a normal or near-normal CEA pre-surgery (at baseline) have a better prognosis than those with a high baseline level.

CEA may be elevated in other cancers, including pancreas, lung, breast, and ovary. It is more useful in some patients than in others.

While this testing is being done, the patient will be referred for a consultation with a surgeon. If the CT scan, CEA, and liver enzyme test are normal, the surgery will be done with the intention of curing the cancer, i.e., a curative resection. Usually either the right or left half of the colon will be removed along with the blood vessels and lymph nodes in the area. It is particularly important that the resection be large enough to include at least twelve lymph nodes so that the presence or absence of lymph node involvement can be accurately determined. Surgery may be appropriate even if there are liver metastases on the CT scan in order to prevent a complete blockage of flow through the colon (intestinal obstruction). Many colon resections can be done laparoscopically, using a thin scope placed through a small incision, similar to those used in gallbladder surgery. The benefits of laparoscopic surgery include a smaller incision, less pain, and a shorter hospital stay.

After surgery, the stage of the colon cancer[6] will be determined based on the analysis of the tissue removed and the CT scan, or other imaging studies. Staging is with the TNM system, encompassing features of the depth of invasion of the tumor (T), involvement of lymph nodes (N), and metastases (M), if any. The following is a very simplified summary of the stages of colon cancer based on the categories and subcategories of the TNM stages:

STAGES OF COLON CANCER

Stage I The tumor remains below the muscle layer of the colon or invades the muscle layer. No positive lymph nodes or metastases.

Stage II The tumor invades the tissue on top of the muscle layer of the colon, the membrane lining of the abdominal cavity, or adjacent structures. No positive lymph nodes or metastases.

Stage III Any depth of invasion. One or more positive lymph nodes. No metastases.

Stage IV Any depth of invasion. Any number of lymph nodes. Distant metastases present.

Referral to an oncologist will be made in most cases, and the oncologist will take over most of the management at this point. Chemotherapy will often be prescribed, and a detailed discussion of chemotherapy is beyond the scope of this book, as it is rarely, if ever, prescribed by the gastroenterologist. It is important to note, however, that chemotherapy has become more effective and less toxic over the years, though significant side effects remain.

There are several forms of chemotherapy:

- **Adjuvant chemotherapy** is given to patients who have had a potentially curative resection with or without positive lymph nodes. The purpose of adjuvant chemotherapy is to destroy small collections of cancer cells that remain after surgery, resulting in a higher cure rate.
- **Neo-adjuvant chemotherapy** is given *before* surgery in order to shrink the tumor and make the resection easier and more likely to be successful. It is used in larger rectal tumors, especially if they are very low (distal) in the rectum.
- **Palliative chemotherapy** is given to patients with stage IV (metastatic) colon cancer and can prolong survival. It is not given with the intention to cure.

Surgery for one or a few metastases to the lungs or liver can be effective; the survival may increase and some cures may result. All of these decisions are individualized and require expert medical judgment.

Colonoscopy is recommended at one year after surgical resection, with subsequent colonoscopies at three and five years, respectively, if nothing is found on the preceding colonoscopy.

RECENT COLON CANCER SURVIVAL STATISTICS[7]

- For patients diagnosed in 2003–2009, the overall five-year survival was 65 percent.
- In rectal cancer and distal (left-sided) colon cancer, patients under age sixty-five have a five-year survival of 69 percent, versus 62 percent in patients age sixty-five or older. The five-year survival in proximal colon cancer is 65 percent in both groups.
- The five-year survival for early stage (I or II) colon cancer is 90 percent, but only 40 percent of colon cancers are stage I or II at the time of initial diagnosis.
- The five-year survival for stage III is 70 percent and only 12.5 percent for stage IV.
- African Americans have lower survival rates at all stages. This difference is thought to be a result of reduced access to screening and effective treatment, and the effects of coexisting medical conditions.
- Adjuvant chemotherapy significantly improves survival for both African American and Caucasian patients with stage III colon cancer.

Rectal Cancer

Rectal cancer is diagnosed similarly to colon cancer, and surgery is the definitive treatment. There are some important differences in the behavior and treatment of rectal cancer as compared with colon cancer:[8]

- Rectal cancer is more likely to recur locally, at the original site or the anastomosis (site of surgical reconnection).
- Rectal cancer that recurs is less likely to be resectable (able to be removed surgically) than colon cancer.
- Neoadjuvant chemotherapy and radiation therapy are often recommended, especially for more advanced cancers.

CASE REPORT: A CLOSE CALL

Mildred S. had her first screening colonoscopy at age sixty-four, well after the recommended age of fifty. Dr. Fioretti performed the procedure, and she removed a 10-millimeter adenoma. She recommended a three-year follow-up colonoscopy and also advised Mildred to quit smoking. Mildred did not call the office to schedule the colonoscopy, despite the recall letters sent to her and to her primary care physician.

Mildred came back 7½ years later. She told Dr. Fioretti that her family doctor found blood in the stool. Mildred had not seen any blood but admitted that she didn't look too carefully. A note from the family doctor indicated that he was requesting evaluation for a positive stool for occult blood, upper abdominal pain, and a twenty-pound weight loss over the last four months. Dr. Fioretti recommended colonoscopy. Dr. Fioretti asked, "Did you get any letters from our office about coming in sooner for your colonoscopy?"

"Yes, I did."

"And why haven't we heard from you?"

"I just didn't want to drink that stuff."

The colonoscopy showed a large mass in the proximal transverse colon. The mass occluded the lumen of the colon, and the scope could not advance farther. Mildred was referred to a surgeon and had a right colon resection. She was a stage II, and all of her lymph nodes were negative. However, her baseline CEA was elevated, and her oncologist recommended adjuvant chemotherapy. She tolerated this well, and the CEA returned to normal.

Follow-up colonoscopies were negative, and she has remained in complete remission for more than five years. She has continued to smoke cigarettes.

TAKE-HOME MESSAGES

- If you are diagnosed with colon cancer, try to maintain a positive attitude. Many cancers are curable and proper treatment can prolong life at any stage.
- Initially you will need a CT scan, blood tests, and usually a surgical consultation.
- Some colon resections can be done through a laparoscope, with the advantages of less post-operative pain and a shorter hospital stay.
- After surgery, the tumor will be staged, based on the depth of invasion, involvement of lymph nodes in the area, and metastases.
- An oncologist will usually guide the care at this point.
- Follow-up colonoscopies are very important.

8

Diverticulosis and Diverticulitis

Colon polyps and cancer are not the only problems of the lower GI tract. Diverticulitis is among the most common causes of abdominal pain that may be severe enough to require hospitalization. It involves infection or inflammation of small outpouchings of the colon called diverticula. The standard terms describing diverticular disease are summarized below.

DIVERTICULAR DICTIONARY

Diverticula	Two or more outpouchings in the intestinal tract, most commonly in the colon
Diverticular	Characterized by diverticulosis, as in diverticular disease or diverticular abscess
Diverticulitis	An infection or inflammation of a diverticulum or diverticula
Diverticulosis	The presence of diverticula
Diverticulum	A single outpouching in the intestinal tract

DIVERTICULITIS AND DIVERTICULOSIS

Diverticulosis denotes the presence of outpouchings on the inside of the colon (see figure 8.1). A single pouch is called a *diverticulum* (the plural being *diverticula*). Diverticula are seen as craters in the lining of the colon during colonoscopy, but would be seen as outpouchings at surgery, or on an X-ray of the colon when the colon is filled with contrast. Diverticula can occur in other parts of the GI tract, but in the colon they tend to occur in areas where

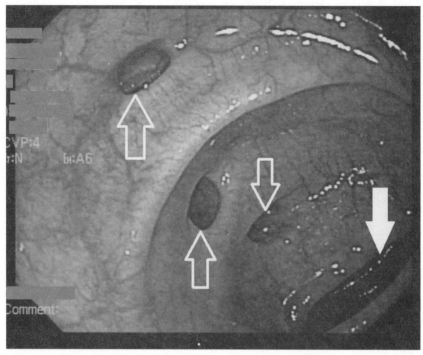

Figure 8.1.   Diverticulosis as seen at colonoscopy. The diverticula are seen as craters (open arrows). The closed arrow points to the lumen, the channel or opening of the colon.
Source: David M. Novick, *Diverticulosis*, July 2016.

a blood vessel penetrates the muscle layer of the colon. Diverticula have thin walls and lack the usual muscular layer.

Diverticulosis is common in the United States and other developed countries. It becomes more likely with increasing age, and most people with diverticulosis are middle-aged or elderly. About 50 percent of Americans have it by age fifty. The number of diverticula also increases with age. In the West, most diverticula are seen in the left colon, but in Asia right colon diverticulosis predominates.[1] Diverticulosis usually has no symptoms. Problems occur when a diverticulum bleeds or becomes infected. The latter situation is called *diverticulitis*.

The cause of diverticulosis is unknown. The most promising theory is that it results from abnormal contractions, which lead to increased pressure within the colon.[2] The increased pressure leads to outpouchings in areas of weakness in the colon. Early studies suggest a role of insufficient fiber in the diet over many years or decades, and a high-fiber diet is often recommended. While not proven to prevent further development of diverticula, or of diverticulitis, a high-fiber diet has other benefits, including more regular stools and lower cholesterol levels. Many people believe that popcorn, nuts, or foods with seeds should be avoided in diverticulosis because they might become packed into a diverticulum causing an obstruction or infection. However, studies have failed to show any benefit in restricting these foods,[3] although it is probably best to avoid eating a two-liter container of popcorn in one sitting.

Diverticulitis is characterized by moderate to severe pain in the left lower abdomen. This may be accompanied by fever, diarrhea, constipation, nausea, and vomiting. The diagnosis is made from typical signs and symptoms, as well as CT scan results showing inflammation in the left colon. Diverticulitis is sometimes called "left-sided appendicitis" (appendicitis typically presents with pain in the right lower abdomen). Most cases can be treated with oral antibiotics in outpatient settings, but severe cases may require hospitalization and IV antibiotics. Diverticulitis can be complicated by spontaneous bowel perforation or the formation of an abscess. The tear in the colon is treated surgically, while the abscess is drained, most commonly by insertion of a drainage tube using CT scanning for correct placement.

A newer concept is that diverticulitis can be chronic. Some cases of diverticulitis more closely resemble a chronic inflammatory condition rather than an acute infection, and antibiotics are less beneficial than previously thought.[4]

It was traditionally taught that about 10–25 percent of patients with diverticulosis will ever develop diverticulitis. A recent study from the Veterans Affairs Healthcare System revealed that in a large group of people who had diverticulosis found incidentally on colonoscopy and were followed for eleven years, only 4.3 percent developed diverticulitis.[5] Younger patients had a higher risk. The risk of diverticulitis increases with smoking and obesity, and decreases with regular physical activity.[6] Diverticulitis can occur more than once. Surgery has often been recommended for patients with three or more cases of diverticulitis, but a more recent concept is that surgery to prevent diverticulitis may not be necessary unless complications have occurred. Further research is needed. Elective (non-emergency) surgery for diverticulitis is very safe, and many patients will benefit. However, 5–25 percent of patients who undergo such surgery will not have symptom relief.[7]

Bleeding is another serious complication of diverticulosis. The risk of bleeding is increased in patients who take non-steroidal anti-inflammatory drugs (NSAIDs),[8] examples of which are ibuprofen and naproxen. Diverticular bleeding is typically painless, large volume, and bright red. The bleeding is usually perceived as severe, leading to a visit to the emergency room. When patients are hospitalized for lower GI bleeding, a colonoscopy is often done to try to identify the cause and the exact location of the bleeding. If the bleeding is a result of diverticulosis, it is usually not possible to identify the specific site of bleeding because the large amount of blood obscures too many details. If the bleeding is rapid enough, the site can be identified by X-rays during an injection of contrast into the vascular system. A substance can then be injected into the specific vessel to stop the bleeding. Most episodes of diverticular bleeding stop on their own, and surgery is rarely needed.

TAKE-HOME MESSAGES

- Diverticulosis is common, but causes no difficulty in 85 percent or more of those with this condition.
- People with diverticulosis do not need to restrict nuts or vegetables with seeds.
- Diverticulitis is a potentially serious condition that usually presents itself with pain in the left lower abdomen.
- Diverticulitis may not always require antibiotics, but it is standard practice in many areas to prescribe them.

9

Irritable Bowel Syndrome

IRRITABLE BOWEL SYNDROME

This chapter will cover irritable bowel syndrome (IBS), a disorder that affects 10–15 percent of adults. IBS is not limited to the colon but has similar symptoms to other colon problems.

Irritable bowel syndrome is the most common bowel disorder and the second most prevalent medical reason, after the common cold, for absence from work. It is a functional disorder, i.e., a condition in which the intestinal tract is normal when examined, even under a microscope, but bodily processes are abnormal. IBS is manifested by various combinations of abdominal pain, constipation, and diarrhea. A change in the bowel pattern is usually noted when the symptoms begin.[1] Diarrhea, alternating with constipation, is a frequent pattern that occurs with IBS. Bloating is a typical complaint. IBS is common in young adults, and women are affected more than men. Variants of IBS include constipation-predominant, diarrhea-predominant, and mixed (alternating diarrhea and constipation).

The abdominal pain is typically crampy, intermittent, and frequently relieved by a bowel movement.[2] Appetite and weight are unchanged. The pain does not become progressively worse over time, and does not awaken the patient from sleep. It is not associated with bleeding, though mucus may be present in the stool. The constipation is sometimes described as pellet-like stools, and may alternate with diarrhea or normal stools. The diarrhea is often small volume and associated with cramps and a sense of incomplete evacuation.

ALARM SYMPTOMS

If these symptoms are present, it may not be IBS. Further evaluation is required.

- Weight loss
- Gastrointestinal bleeding
- Awakening from sleep with pain or diarrhea
- Iron deficiency anemia

There is no specific test to diagnose IBS and no underlying disorder to treat. Laboratory tests, imaging (such as CT scans and small-bowel X-rays), esophagogastroduodenoscopy, colonoscopy, and biopsies are normal in patients with IBS. Such testing is often done to rule out other conditions, including celiac disease, thyroid problems, ulcerative colitis, or Crohn's disease. Some cases are triggered by gastroenteritis or other acute GI infections. IBS is often associated with anxiety and stress, and a history of abuse is not uncommon. It does not progress to Crohn's disease, ulcerative colitis, cancer, or any other condition.

Treatment of IBS can be divided into three main categories: diet, lifestyle, and medications. People with IBS often make dietary changes on their own, before consulting a physician or a dietitian. There are several things to keep in mind when so doing. First, symptoms of IBS may be related to meals eaten before the most recent one. Keeping a **food and symptom diary** may help you see an association between diet and symptoms. Second, if you eliminate too many foods, your remaining diet may be deficient or unbalanced. Third, IBS and its symptoms overlap with other common disorders, including *lactose intolerance* and *celiac disease*. Eliminating dairy products is generally of little benefit in IBS, but can be very beneficial in lactose intolerance, a disorder in which the small intestine cannot break down lactose.[3] A gluten-free diet is widely used without consultation but will cause laboratory tests and biopsies for celiac disease to become negative, making the diagnosis much more difficult (see chapter 15, "Disorders of the Stomach and Small Intestine, Including Celiac Disease").

A major advance in the dietary treatment of IBS is the low-FODMAP diet.[4] FODMAPs are short-chain carbohydrates (sugars) that are poorly absorbed into the body. Remaining too long in the small intestine, they pull excess water into the bowel by osmosis. Also, they are fermented by bowel bacteria, and the by-products of this fermentation include various gases.[5] The increased fluid and gas in the intestinal tract can cause pain and bloating in patients with IBS, who are more sensitive to such changes than are others. People without IBS usually have no problem with these foods.

FODMAP is an acronym for fermentable oligosaccharides, disaccharides, monosaccharides, and polyols. See glossary for details.

In patients with IBS, controlled studies have shown improvement in symptoms with a low-FODMAP diet.[6] However, the diet is quite complex as it restricts a large number of foods. Many FODMAP-containing foods are "natural" and considered to be healthy, such as apples, mangos, peaches, pears, cauliflower, garlic, onion, cow or goat milk, chickpeas, lentils, rye, and wheat. The list is so extensive that **consultation with a dietitian is strongly recommended** before starting a low-FODMAP diet in order to ensure that the remaining diet is nutritionally sound.[7] Also, patients have pointed out that all of the food lists for the low-FODMAP diet are different. To address this and to give you an idea of the diet, I have devised the Consensus FODMAP Food Lists (see tables 9.1 and 9.2 below), which are shorter lists showing the most commonly cited high- and low-FODMAP foods. Table 9.1 shows high-FODMAP foods that should be avoided in the low-FODMAP diet, and table 9.2 shows low-FODMAP foods that may be eaten. Keep in mind that due to the enormous variety of available foods, this list should be considered basic and not comprehensive—hence the need for a dietitian. Also, it is critical to check ingredients as FODMAP-containing foods may be additives.

Table 9.1   Foods That Should be *Avoided* in the Low-FODMAP diet

Consensus High-FODMAP Food List
To be **avoided** in low-FODMAP diet for IBS.
Dietitian consultation strongly recommended.

Fruits	*Vegetables*	*Dairy*
Apple, apricot, avocado, blackberry, canned fruit, cherry, lychee, mango, nectarine, peach, pear, plum, prune, watermelon	Artichoke, asparagus, brussel sprout, cauliflower, garlic, leek, mushroom, onion, pea, shallot	Buttermilk, cow milk, cream, custard, goat milk, ice cream, margarine, sheep milk, soft unripe cheese, yogurt (unless lactose-free and without the sweeteners noted below)
Sweeteners	*Legumes*	*Grains*
Fructose, high-fructose corn syrup, honey, inulin, isomalt, maltitol, mannitol, sorbitol, sucralose, xylitol, others ending in -ol	Baked beans, chickpeas, kidney beans, lentils, soybeans	Rye, semolina, wheat *Miscellaneous* Dandelion tea

Table 9.2.   Foods That May Be Eaten in the Low-FODMAP Diet

Consensus Low-FODMAP Food List
May be eaten in low-FODMAP diet for IBS.
Dietitian consultation strongly recommended.

Fruits	*Vegetables*	*Dairy*
Blueberry, cantaloupe, cranberry, grapes, honeydew, kiwi, lemon, lime, mandarin orange, papaya, passion fruit, pineapple, raspberry, strawberry	Bean sprouts, bok choy, carrot, chives, corn,* cucumber, eggplant, ginger, green beans, lettuce, olives, parsnip, potato, spinach (baby), spring onion (green part), squash, sweet potato,* tomato,** turnip, zucchini	Lactose-free milk, lactose-free yogurt, rice milk, some cheeses: brie, camembert, feta, mozzarella, parmesan *Alcohol* Vodka, wine*
Sweeteners	*Protein*	*Grains and Nuts*
Aspartame, glucose, maple syrup, saccharine, sucrose (table sugar) *Miscellaneous* Coffee, herbal tea***	Beef, chicken, eggs, fish, lamb, pork, seafood, tofu, turkey	Gluten-free oats, macadamia nuts, millet, peanuts, pecans, pine nuts, pumpkin seeds, quinoa, rice, sesame seeds, sorghum, sunflower seeds, walnuts

*Limited quantities.
**Not cherry tomatoes.
***Not apple or dandelion tea.

If you wish to start a low-FODMAP diet before consulting a physician or dietitian, a reasonable initial approach is to avoid all of the sweeteners listed in table 9.1. You may be surprised to see how many foods contain these.

After you have responded to the low-FODMAP diet, you do not necessarily have to stay on the same form of it forever. The initial goal is to understand how your body responds to elimination of FODMAP-containing foods. Working with your dietitian, you may gradually reintroduce small quantities of selected restricted foods and assess the response.

Traditionally, a high-fiber diet has been recommended for IBS, but results are variable. Many patients complain of increased gas with a high-fiber diet or fiber supplements, as most but not all fiber, whether in food or supplements, undergoes fermentation (see chapter 19, "Healthy Eating"). Avoiding gas-producing foods such as beans, celery, cabbage, and all carbonated drinks is a simple measure that may help.

Lifestyle changes consist of exercise and stress reduction. Most Americans are too sedentary. Regular walking, in addition to walking at work or with a dog, is a good place to start. Advancing to more vigorous exercise may be more beneficial, but if you have underlying health problems it is best to consult your primary care physician before starting. If anxiety or depression is present, professional help and the right combination of counseling, therapy, medications, and exercise can be very effective. Remember that although IBS can be very stressful and unpleasant, it is a medical problem and not psychological or psychosomatic. For non-pharmacologic stress reduction, consider one or more of the following: yoga, meditation, relaxation exercises, reading the Scripture of your choice, stretching, massage, and heat treatments.

Many medications are used for IBS (table 9.3). Most are effective for one symptom only. Consult your physician to see which, if any, is best for you.

Table 9.3. Medications for Irritable Bowel Syndrome (IBS)

	Constipation	Diarrhea	Pain
Over the counter	Fiber supplements (psyllium, bran, others), polyethylene glycol (MiraLAX, GlycoLax, others), laxatives, probiotics	Loperamide (Imodium), probiotics	Acetaminophen. Do not take aspirin or anti-inflammatory drugs for abdominal pain, except on your doctor's advice.
Prescription	Lubiprostone (Amitiza), linaclotide (Linzess), lactulose	Cholestyramine, rifaximin (Xyfaxan), diphenoxylate/atropine (Lomotil), eluxadoline (Viberzi)	Antispasmodics (dicyclomine, hyosciamine, others), amitriptyline

A few comments on medications: Constipation is usually treated initially with dietary changes, fiber supplements, or polyethylene glycol (also discussed in chapter 1, "Preparing for Colonoscopy"). Lubiprostone and Linaclotide have been very effective in some patients. Cholestyramine may work for diarrhea, especially in people who have had their gallbladder removed, but it needs to be taken apart from certain other medications, especially thyroid supplements. Rifaximin has had some success in studies but is expensive. While amitriptyline is an antidepressant, it is used here in low doses as a pain modulator. Eluxadoline should be used with caution in people in whom the gallbladder has been removed. It should not be used in patients with bile duct disorders, alcohol abuse, severe liver disease, or previous pancreatitis, or in those drinking more than three alcoholic drinks per day. It is a controlled substance, on Schedule IV of the Controlled

Substances Act, and it can produce euphoria, although this is rare in standard doses in IBS patients who are not "recreational opioid-experienced individuals."[8] Diphenoxylate/atropine is a Schedule V controlled substance.

What about probiotics? Probiotics are "good bacteria" or other microorganisms that are taken in supplements or food and intended to maintain or restore normal bowel function (see also chapter 19). There are many products, but only a few high-quality studies. Due to the tremendous interest in intestinal bacteria, often referred to as the microbiome or microbiota (see chapter 19), advances in our knowledge in this area are anticipated in the next decade. If you take probiotics, remember the following:

- Choose a product with several strains of bacteria, rather than one.
- Yogurt and kefir are good sources of probiotics from food.
- Change probiotics every three to six months.
- If you take drugs that suppress the immune system, or have a disease that does this, do not take probiotics unless approved by your physician.

TAKE-HOME MESSAGES

- IBS is a medical disorder with no specific abnormality on examination, blood tests, or biopsies. It is referred to as a functional disorder.
- IBS symptoms are abdominal pain, bloating, diarrhea, and/or constipation. Alternating diarrhea and constipation is typical of IBS. Bleeding, weight loss, or waking up at night because of symptoms (alarm symptoms) should suggest other diagnoses.
- Treatments for IBS include diet, lifestyle changes, and medications.
- Foods that are "natural" and "organic" may cause symptoms in people with IBS. In IBS, "an apple a day makes your gut cry foul play." Many fruits, vegetables, legumes, dairy products, and sweeteners contain FODMAPs, and these can be poorly tolerated in IBS.
- A low-FODMAP diet can be helpful, but is best approached with guidance from a dietitian.

10

Crohn's Disease and Ulcerative Colitis (Inflammatory Bowel Disease)

Crohn's disease and ulcerative colitis are characterized by inflammation of the GI tract and are collectively known as inflammatory bowel disease. They have many similarities and differences. There is a wide spectrum of clinical manifestations, ranging from mild to severe. These disorders are much less common than irritable bowel syndrome. The cause is unknown, and while they can be treated, in most cases they cannot be cured.

Both diseases are thought of as autoimmune diseases, meaning that the patient's immune system is reacting against his or her own body tissues—in this case, those of the GI tract. The target to which the immune system is reacting is not known. Some investigators have suspected that the process starts as a food allergy, and the immune reaction against the food somehow transfers to the bowel wall. Infection with a surreptitious bacteria or virus has long been suspected, but never proven. Genetic factors play a role, as these diseases are more common in family members than in the general population. As in irritable bowel syndrome, an acute GI infection sometimes triggers or unmasks inflammatory bowel disease. Crohn's disease is more common and more severe in smokers, but cigarette smoking may protect against ulcerative colitis—one of the few diseases for which smoking is "beneficial." Smoking is definitely not recommended in any patient, even in one whose symptoms improve with smoking.

Both disorders are most commonly present in people ages fifteen to forty; some studies have shown a second peak incidence at about age fifty-five to sixty-five. Crohn's disease is slightly more common in females, and ulcerative colitis in males. Both tend to be more common in more northern latitudes.

Ulcerative colitis almost always starts in the rectum and extends into the colon from there. Its area of involvement is continuous, and it does not affect other parts of the GI tract. Surgical specimens show that the inflammation in ulcerative colitis is limited to the innermost layer (covering the walls of the lumen) of the rectum and colon. Crohn's disease, on the other hand, can involve any part of the GI tract, from the mouth to the anus, though it is most common in the colon and last part of the small intestine (terminal ileum). It is not continuous and can have "skip areas" in which areas of normal bowel exist in between areas affected by Crohn's disease. The rectum is uninvolved in about half of the patients with Crohn's disease. The inflammation in Crohn's disease extends throughout all of the layers of the intestine. This deeper, more extensive inflammation leads to thickening of the bowel and, in some cases, strictures (areas of narrowing) or even bowel obstruction. It may also explain the findings in Crohn's disease of fistulas (abnormal connections) between loops of bowel, from bowel to skin, or from bowel to other sites such as the urinary tract.

The cardinal symptom of ulcerative colitis is small-volume diarrhea. Multiple episodes, sometimes ten to fifteen per day, are common. The diarrhea is associated with bleeding, mucus in the stool, urgency, and/or tenesmus (painful straining at stool). Fever, anemia, and weight loss may occur. Toxic megacolon, a dilation of the colon with severe symptoms, is rare but may necessitate emergency surgery. Arthritis, skin disorders, certain eye problems, and liver abnormalities may be associated with either ulcerative colitis or Crohn's disease.

Crohn's disease is most commonly manifested by fatigue, abdominal pain, weight loss, and diarrhea. Bleeding may be present, but is less common than in ulcerative colitis. Fistulas and perianal disease are typical of Crohn's disease. The perianal problems include pain, fistulas, abscess, anal fissure (see chapter 12, "Hemorrhoids"), and persistent drainage. Kidney stones are linked with this disorder. Table 10.1 compares the features of Crohn's disease and ulcerative colitis.

The diagnosis is derived from data obtained by the history, physical examination, laboratory tests, imaging, colonoscopy, biopsy, and occasionally capsule endoscopy of the small intestine. Some patients (less than 10 percent) with disease only in the colon can be difficult to classify as having ulcerative colitis or Crohn's disease and are considered "indeterminate."

Table 10.1. Comparison of Crohn's Disease and Ulcerative Colitis*

	Crohn's Disease	*Ulcerative Colitis*
Suggestive symptoms	• Abdominal pain, especially right lower abdomen	• Bloody diarrhea • Rectal pain • Tenesmus
Associated smoking status**	• Smoker	• Non-smoker • Former smoker
Area of GI tract involvement	• Any part of the GI tract	• Colon only*** • Starts in rectum and extends proximally
Depth of involvement	All layers of intestine	Innermost layer only
Skip areas	Yes	No
Fistula, stricture, abscess	Yes	No

*No laboratory test can distinguish these two entities with certainty.
**These are the usual relationships. Exceptions may occur.
***The terminal ileum can show inflammation in ulcerative colitis. This is known as "backwash ileitis" and is more common when the entire colon is involved with ulcerative colitis.

TREATMENT OF INFLAMMATORY BOWEL DISEASE

There are many medications used for inflammatory bowel disease:

- **Aminosalycilates** (sulfasalazine, mesalamine, balsalazide). These medications contain a compound closely related to aspirin. They are used in mild to moderate ulcerative colitis to induce remission (to treat and suppress the symptoms) and to prevent relapses. Aminosalycilates are not effective in Crohn's disease. Sulfasalazine is the least expensive because it has been used for decades and is available as a generic. It has significantly more side effects than mesalamine because it contains a sulfa component in addition to the aspirin-like compound. Mesalamine and balsalazide are newer aminosalycilates. Mesalamine comes in several delayed-release formulations, allowing it to reach much, or all, of the colon if given orally. There are also liquid or solid forms for rectal insertion. Oral and rectal mesalamine can be used together. Mesalamine and balsalazide are generally well tolerated, although nausea, vomiting, joint pains, and other side effects may occur. Rarely, serious toxicity may occur, e.g., liver or kidney injury, inflammation in or around the heart, or major changes in blood counts. It is important to monitor for kidney injury if these drugs are used long term.
- **Antibiotics**. They may help for mild Crohn's disease and in people with Crohn's disease who have fistulas. Ciprofloxacin, metronidazole, or rifaximin are most commonly used. Improvements are usually short term.

- **Oral corticosteroids** (prednisone). Prednisone is given orally for both Crohn's disease and ulcerative colitis, and is commonly used for flare-ups. In most patients, prednisone will induce a partial or complete remission (resolution of symptoms), but symptoms usually recur shortly after prednisone has been stopped. Prednisone and other corticosteroids are often referred to as "steroids," but they are not the type that some athletes and bodybuilders use.

WARNING: DO NOT STOP PREDNISONE ABRUPTLY

Unless used for one to two weeks only, prednisone and similar corticosteroid drugs must not be stopped abruptly. They should be slowly tapered with the dose reduced a little at a time, according to your doctor's instructions.

- **Intravenous corticosteroids** (hydrocortisone, methylprednisolone) are used for severe flare-ups that require hospitalization; after improvement, the patient will be transitioned to prednisone. All corticosteroids have serious side effects if taken long term, and most gastroenterologists try very hard not to prescribe them for longer than four weeks. The repeated need for corticosteroids to suppress flare-ups is an indicator that immunosuppressive or biologic drugs are necessary.

STEROID SIDE EFFECTS

- Weight gain
- Fluid retention
- Rounded face
- Thinning of bones (osteoporosis)
- Cataracts
- Elevated blood sugar
- Serious hip damage (aseptic necrosis)
- Elevated cholesterol
- Mental status changes such as agitation, anxiety, and excessive energy
- Insomnia
- Elevated blood pressure
- Increased risk of infection

- **Budesonide** is a corticosteroid that is less well absorbed into the body from the GI tract, resulting in more of the drug staying in the GI tract, where it can be useful for mild to moderate Crohn's disease involving the terminal ileum or right colon. An extended-release form, UCERIS, can be used for ulcerative colitis. Budesonide has steroid side effects and is not recommended for maintenance treatment beyond a few months. It interacts with several drugs, so be sure to ask your doctor about this. Of particular note, drugs that block stomach acid (see chapter 15, "Disorders of the Stomach and Small Intestine, Including Celiac Disease") may alter the absorption of budesonide.

- **Immunomodulators** (azathioprine, 6-mercaptopurine [6-MP]; also referred to as immunosuppressive drugs) are excellent medications for maintaining remission of moderate to severe Crohn's disease or ulcerative colitis. They are not effective in inducing remission and therefore are often used with corticosteroids. Their full effect may not be seen for three to six months. Although they may have significant side effects, they are very well tolerated by most patients. Methotrexate is another immunomodulator that is used infrequently, because of possible liver injury, and only for Crohn's disease.

SIDE EFFECTS OF AZATHIOPRINE OR 6-MP

- Decreased white cell count*
- Liver injury*
- Decreased platelet count*
- Inflammation of pancreas (pancreatitis)
- Anemia*
- Nausea and vomiting
- Increased risk of infection
- Rash
- A small increase in certain cancers: lymphoma and skin cancers (not melanoma)
- Fever

*Because of these side effects, monitoring blood counts and liver tests is an important part of the management of patients on azathioprine or 6-MP.

- **Biologic drugs** are manufactured in a biological system, such as a bacteria or cell culture, rather than by a chemical process. The first-generation biologic drugs used in inflammatory bowel disease are inhibitors of tumor necrosis factor (TNF), a protein that promotes acute inflammation. Blocking TNF suppresses the immune response and reduces inflammation. They are given intravenously or by subcutaneous (under the skin) injection. Other types of biologic drugs are available or in clinical trials, and a tremendous expansion of the menu of biologic drugs for the treatment of inflammatory bowel disease is anticipated.

BIOLOGIC DRUGS FOR INFLAMMATORY BOWEL DISEASE

TNF Inhibitors for Crohn's Disease

- Infliximab (Remicade)
- Adalimumab (HUMIRA)
- Certolizumab pegol (CIMZIA)

TNF Inhibitors for Ulcerative Colitis

- Infliximab (Remicade)
- Adalimumab (HUMIRA)
- Golimumab (Simponi)

Integrin Inhibitor

- Vedolizumab (ENTYVIO)

Interleukin-12 and -23 Inhibitor for Crohn's Disease

- Ustekinumab (STELARA)

Biologic drugs are very effective in moderate to severe Crohn's disease or ulcerative colitis, and they are becoming the treatment of choice for these patients. They are particularly helpful in Crohn's disease with a fistula formation. In general, the first TNF inhibitor used in treatment will be the most effective, but occasionally a patient may develop an adverse effect or loss of effect of the drug and may respond well to another TNF inhibitor. The TNF inhibitors are generally well tolerated, but serious adverse effects may occur. These drugs are very expensive but are usually covered by insurance. Financial assistance from the pharmaceutical companies may also be available.

Biologic drugs are foreign substances, and the body can reject them by making antibodies. Antibodies to a biologic drug can render it ineffective. When a patient does not respond to a biologic or stops responding, testing for antibodies can be very important; if antibodies are detected, then it is necessary to change to a different biologic. Testing for blood levels of biologic drugs, to be sure that a sufficient amount of drug is in the blood and reaching the affected areas, can also be critical. If the blood level is too low, but no antibodies are present, either the dose can be increased or the dosing interval can be shortened. At this time, testing for blood levels and antibodies is commercially available for infliximab and adalimumab.

SIDE EFFECTS OF TNF INHIBITORS

- Reactivation of tuberculosis
- Severe fungal infection
- Bacterial infection
- Reactivation of hepatitis B
- Virus infection
- Infusion reactions
- Liver injury
- Psoriasis
- Decreases in blood counts
- Increased risk of cancer, including lymphoma and skin cancers

Vedolizumab is a biologic that blocks inflammation specifically in the GI tract. It can induce and maintain remission and reduce the use of corticosteroids in moderate to severe Crohn's disease and ulcerative colitis.[1,2] Patients who have previously been treated with anti-TNF drugs can respond to vedolizumab, but do so less often than those not previously treated. Vedolizumab is more effective in ulcerative colitis than Crohn's disease.[3] It is given by intravenous infusion. Side effects include allergic reactions, colds and respiratory infections, liver injury, headache, and rash.

HOW IS VEDOLIZUMAB GUT SPECIFIC?

Vedolizumab is a biologic drug that blocks inflammation within the GI tract. This drug interferes with the normal biologic system that regulates the migration of a particular type of white blood cell, the effector T lymphocyte, from the bloodstream into tissues at the site of injury or infection. In order to reach such a site, the T lymphocyte must attach to the blood vessel wall and then migrate through it. One group of molecules that facilitates this migration, the integrins, resides on the surface of T lymphocytes. Integrins stop the T lymphocyte from traveling along the surface of the blood vessel and initiate its transit through the vessel wall into the tissue. Integrins carry out this function by interacting with molecules that can appear on blood vessels called adhesion molecules.[4]

One type of integrin, α4β7, is seen on T lymphocytes that reside in and around the GI tract. It interacts with a molecule, mucosal addressin cell adhesion molecule 1, or MAdCAM-1, that resides on blood vessels in the small intestine and colon.[5] This interaction is "gut specific" as it is involved with T lymphocyte migration only in the GI tract and not in other tissues.[6] Vedolizumab is a manufactured protein that interferes with the interaction of integrin α4β7 with MAdCAM-1, decreasing the ability of the T lymphocytes to migrate through the vessel wall into the tissue. It thus reduces GI tract inflammation but not inflammation in other sites.

Given the high cost of biologic drugs ($1,078–$5,000 per dose),[7] the question of less expensive generics is often raised. Biologic drugs are large, complex molecules manufactured in biologic systems. If another company produces the drug, differences from the original version in both the manufacturing process and the final drug that results are inevitable. It is possible, however, to make biosimilars, i.e., biologic drugs that have the same beneficial and adverse effects as the original. In April 2016, the Food and Drug Administration approved infliximab-dyyb (Inflectra), the first biosimilar for the treatment of inflammatory bowel disease.[8] Many more biosimilars are anticipated, but whether they result in cost savings remains to be seen.

Treatment regimens can be divided into "step-up" or "top-down." The step-up approach consists of starting with the safest drug, albeit one with lower efficacy. Accordingly, a patient with mild ulcerative colitis might be started on aminosalicylates.[9] The top-down approach, in contrast, would utilize the most effective drug, usually a biologic, early in the course. Biologic drugs are generally more effective as single agents than immunomodulators, and at this writing are more likely to be preferred as the initial treatment for moderate to severe disease. Biologic drugs may be started during or immediately after a course of corticosteroids. Immunomodulators are more likely to be used in combination with biologics when symptoms persist.

Treatment selection is based on the severity of the disease, previous treatments used, and the willingness of the patient to risk drug toxicity. Expert medical judgment is required. Corticosteroids should be used as a short-term intervention, not as maintenance drugs—they are ineffective long term and have numerous side effects. Patients may be asked to sign a consent form outlining the toxicities before starting corticosteroids, immunomodulators, or biologics. Before starting biologic drugs, it is essential to exclude infection, both active, clinically apparent infections and past infections that could reactivate, including tuberculosis and hepatitis B. Also, any needed live vaccines such as that for herpes zoster, shingles (ZOSTAVAX), or influenza (FluMist) must be administered before starting therapy. Check with your doctor to see how soon biologics can be started after a live vaccine.

One treatment that cannot be recommended at this time—though it may well be indicated in the future—is stool transplantation, also known as fecal microbiota transplantation. This involves transferring normal stool from a healthy donor in order to restore the normal bowel bacteria, which may be out of balance in Crohn's disease or ulcerative colitis. The stool suspension can be given through a tube or scope through the mouth into the stomach or small intestine, or through a scope in the rectum. Although very effective in *Clostridium difficile* infection (see chapter 11, "Clostridium difficile Infection, or C-diff"), it has not been adequately studied in inflammatory bowel disease. Some patients are nevertheless doing fecal transplants at home, using guidance from the Internet rather than a doctor or other medical professional, and there have been a few reports of transmission of serious infections.

Surgery to remove the involved area of the small or large intestine is usually a last resort for patients who do not respond well to medical therapy. Surgery can be very effective in some. In Crohn's disease, the inflammation often recurs after surgery at the site of the anastomosis (where the intestine is reconnected after a portion has been surgically removed). Ulcerative colitis can be cured with surgery, but often this entails removing the entire colon, including the rectum. Creation of a pouch using the small intestine is possible for some patients, allowing defecation in the normal way. Other patients may need an ostomy, which is a surgical connection between the intestine and the skin. A colostomy is a connection from the colon to the skin; an ileostomy is one from the ileum, the last part of the small bowel, to the skin. A bag will be worn over the stoma, or opening of the ostomy.

CAN I LIVE WITH "THE BAG"?

It is remarkable how well people can adapt to having a colostomy or ileostomy. The modern equipment makes it easier than in the past. There are several good books on living with an ostomy. Brenda Elsagher has written several, including one that discusses sex after an ostomy.[10,11]

Successful pregnancy is possible in patients with inflammatory bowel disease. The management is complex, but the first principle is **the health of the mother should be maintained**, even if this means continuing prescribed medications during pregnancy. A detailed discussion between the patient and gastroenterologist is essential. Stopping drugs on your own if you are, or might be, pregnant and not following up with your physician is not advisable and can lead to worse outcomes than necessary. A much better approach is to check with your gastroenterologist regarding the best time to start trying to have a baby, especially if your disease is not completely under control.

COLON CANCER AND SURVEILLANCE COLONOSCOPY IN INFLAMMATORY BOWEL DISEASE

The risk of colon cancer is increased in both Crohn's disease and ulcerative colitis. Several factors augment the risk of colon cancer in patients with these conditions:

- Long duration of disease
- Involvement of most or all of the colon
- Severe inflammation
- Family history of colon cancer
- Onset of disease at a young age
- Strictures (areas of narrowing) of the colon
- Primary sclerosing cholangitis, a disease of the bile ducts that is often associated with ulcerative colitis

Surveillance colonoscopy consists of a standard schedule of procedures to look for colon cancer and its forerunner, dysplasia, with the underlying goal of reducing the risk of colon cancer. This is done by taking biopsies (tissue samples) randomly throughout the colon as well as from any suspicious areas, such as polyps or inflamed areas. The biopsies are assessed for dysplasia, a pre-cancerous change consisting of abnormalities in size, shape, or arrangement of the cells or their components.[12] Dysplasia can be low or high grade, with the latter having a higher risk of progression to cancer. If dysplasia is present, the entire colon must be surgically removed unless the dysplasia is limited to a localized structure that can be removed via the colonoscope.[13,14]

There are two innovations that can enhance the detection of dysplasia during colonoscopy. One is chromoendoscopy, in which dye is sprayed through the scope onto the lining of the colon. Another is the use of high-definition scopes and monitors. Both of these techniques make abnormal areas of the colon, which may contain dysplasia, more easily visible to the physician performing the surveillance colonoscopy. These innovations are likely to become the standard of care in the near future.

When should surveillance colonoscopy in inflammatory bowel disease be done? The box shows highlights of the updated guidelines from the American Society for Gastrointestinal Endoscopy (ASGE):

ASGE GUIDELINES FOR SURVEILLANCE COLONOSCOPY IN INFLAMMATORY BOWEL DISEASE[15]

- All patients with ulcerative colitis or Crohn's disease should have a surveillance colonoscopy eight years after the onset of the disease.
- After that, surveillance colonoscopy is done every one to three years, depending on the risk factors for progression to cancer, shown above.
- If ulcerative colitis is limited to the rectum, or rectum and sigmoid, then surveillance is not needed.
- If dysplasia is found in a polyp or other structure that can be completely removed via the colonoscope, then the surveillance colonoscopy is repeated in one to six months, and then in one year.

TAKE-HOME MESSAGES

- Crohn's disease and ulcerative colitis, collectively known as inflammatory bowel disease, have a wide spectrum of clinical manifestations. These disorders can be exceptionally complex, and effective medical care requires excellent communication between physician and patient.
- Inflammatory bowel disease can be treated but is rarely cured.
- Ulcerative colitis starts in the rectum and extends continuously from there. It is limited to the colon. Crohn's disease can affect any part of the GI tract and is typically discontinuous, with skip areas.
- Ulcerative colitis involves only the inner lining of the colon. Crohn's disease extends through the entire thickness of the affected area, leading in some cases to strictures (areas of narrowing) or fistulas (abnormal connections) to skin, urinary tract, or other parts of the bowel.
- There are many medications for inflammatory bowel disease. Expert medical judgment by your gastroenterologist will lead you to the correct treatment.
- Prednisone is very effective in inducing remission of symptoms but because of side effects can only be used for brief intervals. Unless administered for two weeks or less, prednisone must be gradually reduced rather than stopped abruptly.
- If there are repeated flare-ups of Crohn's disease or ulcerative colitis that require the use of prednisone, then the use of immunosuppressive or biologic drugs is usually advisable.
- Immunosuppressive drugs (azathioprine or 6-MP) can often maintain remission of symptoms but are not effective in inducing remission.
- Biologic drugs are very effective in inducing and maintaining remission but have significant side effects and are expensive. The first biologic drug used is often the most effective.
- Successful pregnancy is possible in patients with inflammatory bowel disease. The top priority is maintaining the health of the mother. Do not stop medications on your own.
- Surveillance colonoscopy is recommended for patients with Crohn's disease or ulcerative colitis. The interval depends on the severity and duration of the disease.

11

Clostridium difficile Infection, or C-diff

Clostridium difficile (C-diff) can be considered a disease of technology—infections with C-diff, especially serious ones, are almost always a result of the use of antibiotics. If you are healthy, your hundred trillion normal bacteria, yeasts, and other microbes (collectively known as the microbiome or microbiota), will hold C-diff in check. By decimating the normal bacteria in the colon, antibiotics can allow C-diff to overgrow and cause disease. C-diff causes a particular type of colon inflammation known as pseudomembranous colitis, the main symptom of which is diarrhea. Any antibiotic can trigger C-diff infection, including those used to treat C-diff. The use of multiple antibiotics during hospitalization increases the risk.

In the past fifteen years, the frequency and severity of C-diff infections have been increasing. Contributing factors include the greater use of antibiotics and a more severe and resistant strain of C-diff known as NAP1.[1]

CLOSTRIDIUM DIFFICILE: AN INCREASING PROBLEM[2,3]

- The number of patients discharged from hospitals with a diagnosis of C-diff doubled from 2000 to 2010.
- In 2011, there were approximately 453,000 cases of C-diff in the United States and 29,000 deaths.
- C-diff is the major cause of antibiotic-associated diarrhea in the United States, and the most frequent cause of death from GI infection.

Although otherwise healthy people can contract C-diff, there are known risk factors[4] that include the following:

- Antibiotics, especially prolonged or multiple use
- Recent hospitalization or nursing home stay
- Being over the age of sixty-five
- Proton pump inhibitor (PPI) medications (used for heartburn or reflux)

The C-diff bacteria causes disease because of a toxin that it produces. The toxin damages the cells lining the colon, leading to inflammation and movement of fluid into the lumen of the colon. Some strains do not produce toxin and disease—it's possible that such strains are protective. **C-diff infection can have one or more recurrences and be very difficult to cure in some patients.** It is easily spread by spores, which are small, dormant, and highly resistant forms of C-diff that can survive outside the colon. When they enter the colon, they can grow into an active form. Spores are not eliminated by hand sanitizers or alcohol-based foam; **hand washing for twenty seconds with soap and water** is the best method. Cleaning methods to eliminate spores are discussed later in the chapter.

Watery diarrhea is the main symptom, and it can vary from mild to severe. Patients describe a characteristic foul smell and claim that they can tell when the infection has returned. Abdominal pain, cramps, and fever can be associated with C-diff. Some patients are carriers of C-diff and have no symptoms. If a colonoscopy is done, finding colitis with a pseudomembrane (white or yellow material adhering to the surface of the colon) suggests a C-diff infection, which is also referred to as pseudomembranous colitis. On rare occasions, a very severe, or fulminant, colitis can occur and is manifested by a distended, tender abdomen and a marked elevation of the white blood cell count.

The diagnosis is usually made by stool testing. Colonoscopy is not routinely done but may help if the diagnosis is uncertain.

STOOL TESTING FOR C-DIFF

- Stool testing is only advised when diarrhea is present, or rarely in seriously ill patients with dilated bowel loops on imaging studies.
- If your doctor has ordered stool testing for C-diff, be sure to submit a liquid specimen. A formed stool (one that keeps its shape) may be rejected by the lab.

After treatment of C-diff, stool testing is not recommended unless diarrhea occurs. C-diff may be detectable in carriers without symptoms, who are best not treated. The carrier state of C-diff may be transient, and it very rarely progresses to C-diff with symptoms.[5]

If diarrhea recurs, then stool testing is advisable. Most people with a positive test after treatment of C-diff will have had a relapse of C-diff. Rarely, a patient will develop irritable bowel syndrome (IBS) following an episode of C-diff in a manner similar to other GI infections (see chapter 6, "Colonoscopy: Risks, Alternatives, and Barriers"). Such post-infectious IBS in a carrier of C-diff can be very difficult to distinguish from recurrent C-diff.[6]

About 25 percent of patients have a recurrence of C-diff after the first treatment, and about 50 percent who have had one recurrence will have another. Some second instances of C-diff are reinfection, i.e., reacquisition of C-diff with either the same or a different strain from the original infection, rather than relapse, but testing that would distinguish these two situations is not routinely available.

Risk factors that may lead to a relapse of C-diff include the following:

- Ongoing antibiotic use for other infections
- More severe C-diff at the initial infection
- Age over sixty-five
- Use of PPI medications for reflux; examples are omeprazole, lansoprazole, pantoprazole, and esomeprazole. See chapter 14, "Heartburn and Reflux," for a more complete list.

The medical treatment of C-diff includes antibiotics, probiotics, and infusion of donor feces (also known as fecal microbiota transplant or fecal or stool transplant). The antibiotics for C-diff in common use today are metronidazole, vancomycin, and fidaxomicin.

Metronidazole is used for initial, mild cases of C-diff infection but has become less effective in recent years. It is usually well tolerated but may cause a sensation of "pins and needles" in the hands and feet or a metallic taste in the mouth.

Important: Do not drink alcohol if you are taking metronidazole. It will make you very sick.

Vancomycin is the most commonly prescribed antibiotic for C-diff. It's used for C-diff infections that arise in hospitals, are severe, or recur after previous metronidazole treatment. When used initially, vancomycin is given

---

**TREATMENT OF C-DIFF INFECTION:
MORE THAN ANTIBIOTICS[7,8]**

Although certain antibiotics are needed to cure C-diff, careful attention to the following **in the hospital and in the home** will interrupt its spread and reduce the risk of relapse:

- Stop antibiotic treatment of other infections if possible.
- Follow infection control procedures in hospitals: **all** persons entering hospital rooms of patients with definite or suspected C-diff should wear a disposable gown and gloves.
- Clean stethoscopes.
- Wash hands with **soap and water** for twenty seconds before entering or leaving the hospital room, at home when entering or leaving the bathroom, or before food preparation. *Alcohol-based foams or sanitizers do not kill C-diff spores*. Hand washing should include wrists and between fingers.
- Clean hard surfaces with chlorine bleach diluted 1:10 (one cup bleach and ten cups water). Alternatively, use EPA-registered* sporicides such as Cholox or STERIPLEX, and follow the instructions on the bottle.
- Use towels only once, or use disposable towels.
- Handle soiled linens as little as possible and wash regularly using chlorine bleach.

*EPA is Environmental Protection Agency.

---

orally as a fourteen-day course. Second courses are given for six weeks with gradual dose reduction. This latter regimen includes several weeks of *pulse therapy* in which the vancomycin is given every other day and then every third day.[9] The purpose of pulse therapy is to kill C-diff bacteria that emerge when the spores germinate. If your insurance does not cover vancomycin, it can be expensive: A two-week course of vancomycin 125 mg, four times daily (fifty-six tablets) costs $407.67, and the twelve-week treatment described above costs $1,121,12.[10]

Fidaxomicin is a newer antibiotic that's as effective as vancomycin for treatment of C-diff and may be associated with fewer recurrences. It is more effective than vancomycin when antibiotics for other infections cannot be discontinued.[11] It's given twice daily for a ten-day course and is very expensive; the cost of twenty tablets is $3,494.09.[12]

Probiotics are living microorganisms that are administered for health benefits (see chapter 19, "Healthy Eating"). In C-diff infection, probiotics are taken in the hope that they will restore a normal population of bacteria in the colon that, in turn, will suppress C-diff. For this purpose, they may be most useful before or after taking antibiotics for C-diff or other infections. At this time, we do not know which specific bacteria or combinations of bacteria and other microbes are most effective, and convincing evidence of the effectiveness of probiotics to treat or prevent C-diff is lacking. Nevertheless, it's reasonable to take probiotics after antibiotic treatment for C-diff. Probiotics can be taken as a food (yogurt or kefir) or as a supplement. Probiotics may be dangerous in severely ill patients or those with impaired immune systems; infections from the bacteria in probiotics have been reported in such patients.

When all else fails, C-diff can be treated with fecal microbiota transplant (infusion of donor feces). Stool from a healthy person is administered into the duodenum (beginning of the small intestine) via a tube or scope, or into the colon via a colonoscope. Fecal microbiota transplant delivers an enormous number of normal bacteria to the colon, and these can overwhelm and suppress the C-diff bacteria. In patients with recurrent or refractory C-diff, response rates of 87–92 percent have been reported with fecal microbiota transplant.[13] In a randomized study, fecal microbiota transplant was significantly more effective than vancomycin for the treatment of recurrent C-diff, so much so that the study had to be stopped because of a high relapse rate in the comparison groups but not in the patients receiving fecal transplants.[14] There have been few adverse effects of fecal microbiota transplants for C-diff, with constipation being the most common.

Barriers to the widespread use of fecal transplant for C-diff include the lack of protocols for the procedure at many hospitals and the cost of testing the donor. A stool donor must be checked for a wide variety of infectious diseases, including viral hepatitis and human immunodeficiency virus (HIV). Such testing is not covered by insurance and must be paid for by the patient. A solution to this problem, however, is pre-screened stool that is commercially available. Frozen stool capsules, freeze-dried stool powder, or pre-screened donor enemas are promising agents. A recent study of frozen-and-thawed versus fresh stool for transplantation in recurrent C-diff showed that the frozen stool did not have worse results than the fresh.[15] Several new antibiotics for C-diff are also under study.

TAKE-HOME MESSAGES

- C-diff is a bacterial infection that occurs during or after antibiotic treatment and causes colitis and diarrhea.
- C-diff is increasing in frequency and severity, and it is the major cause of antibiotic-associated diarrhea and the most common cause of death from GI infection in the United States.

- Prolonged or multiple antibiotics increase the risk of C-diff, as does the use of PPI medications for heartburn or reflux. Concern about these risks should engender more thoughtfulness in prescribing but should not limit appropriate use of these medications.
- C-diff is spread by spores (tiny dormant forms of the C-diff bacteria), can recur, and can be very difficult to cure in some patients.
- A limited number of antibiotics is effective against C-diff. When these antibiotics fail, transplant of stool from a healthy donor is often effective.
- The spread of C-diff can be reduced by limiting the use of antibiotics, using infection control procedures at hospitals and nursing homes, hand washing with soap and water for twenty seconds, and cleaning hard surfaces with chlorine bleach or EPA-registered sporicides, diluted 1:10.

12

Hemorrhoids

Everyone has hemorrhoids, which are normal veins in the anal canal. The common use of the term refers to the situation in which these veins enlarge and bleed, itch, or become painful. Hemorrhoids can be external, meaning that they protrude and are visible from the outside. More commonly, they are internal. Hemorrhoids increase in size with increasing age, pregnancy, prolonged sitting, and chronic constipation with frequent straining.

Most people with enlarged hemorrhoids have no symptoms. If you were told that hemorrhoids were seen during your colonoscopy, do not become alarmed. Most hemorrhoids require no treatment.

The initial treatment of mild hemorrhoidal pain or bleeding consists of steps that you can take on your own. They are collectively known as "conservative measures." Hemorrhoids are aggravated by constipation, hard stools, or straining. Taking a stool softener such as docusate (Colace, others) twice a day will help. Fiber supplements such as psyllium or methylcellulose make the stool softer and bulkier, reducing the need to strain. Drinking larger amounts of fluids will help with constipation and will also enhance the effect of fiber supplements by causing the fibers to enlarge. The term "sitz baths" refers to bathing in warm but comfortable water for fifteen minutes. Sitz baths promote healing of the sensitive tissues of the anus. Nothing needs to be added to the water. If you have a sitz bath, be sure to dry the anal area well to prevent a yeast infection.

A variety of over-the-counter medications in the form of suppositories, creams, and ointments are available for anal pain from hemorrhoids. They may contain phenylephrine, which constricts blood vessels and reduces swelling, or soothing substances such as cocoa butter and glycerin that protect the tissues from further irritation.

Depending on the details of your case, your gastroenterologist may prescribe nitroglycerin ointment or rectal creams, foams, or suppositories containing corticosteroids. Nitroglycerin ointment dilates blood vessels and relaxes muscle cells, promoting healing and reducing pain. It is often very effective. Anorectal nitroglycerin is administered at a much lower concentration than that used for heart disease, and to achieve this low concentration the drug is compounded, i.e., created by the pharmacist, at 0.125 percent. Your doctor may prescribe a pea-sized amount of compound nitroglycerin ointment applied to the anus and just inside using a finger cot (a tiny piece of rubber-like material that covers the fingertip). There is also a commercially available form of nitroglycerin ointment that is stronger at 0.4 percent (RECTIV). If you get headaches after using nitroglycerin ointment, you are using too much.

WARNING: If you take sildenafil (Viagra) or similar drugs, you must discontinue them at least twenty-four hours before using nitroglycerin ointment due to a serious drug interaction. Do not restart them until you are no longer using nitroglycerin ointment.

Hydrocortisone, a corticosteroid, is used in many anorectal products, almost all of which require a prescription. Hydrocortisone provides pain relief by reducing inflammation and swelling.

Large hemorrhoidal veins, like all veins, have blood flowing through them. If a clot suddenly forms in a large hemorrhoid, acute severe pain may result. This situation is known as a thrombosed hemorrhoid.

THROMBOSED HEMORRHOID

If you have sudden, severe rectal pain, especially when associated with a new or more severe bulging, contact your doctor immediately. If a patient with a newly formed thrombosed hemorrhoid is seen within forty-eight hours, it's possible for a gastroenterologist or colorectal surgeon to make a small cut in the vein and extract the clot, usually leading to immediate pain relief.

For some anorectal problems, including hemorrhoids, anoscopy may be helpful. This involves insertion of a disposable, lubricated clear plastic scope into the anus to inspect the anal canal and last part of the rectum.

When hemorrhoids cause persistent pain or soiling, a more definitive solution may be sought. Many gastroenterologists perform minimally invasive procedures such as hemorrhoid banding, which does not require a bowel prep or sedation. In this procedure, a disposable, plastic device is used to place a small rubber band around a hemorrhoid that is located far enough into the rectum that doing so will not be painful. The lowest (or most distal) part of the rectum is loaded with nerve endings, and banding there would hurt! Placing a band around a portion of a hemorrhoid leads to a clot forming in the part of the hemorrhoid trapped by the band. In several days, the clot will fall off, leaving an ulcer underneath that will heal with scarring. Such scar tissue will block off the blood vessels and reduce the odds of bleeding. This treatment does not directly affect external hemorrhoids but may help by reducing the blood supply from the internal hemorrhoids that feed the external ones. Other minimally invasive procedures for hemorrhoids that may be performed by gastroenterologists include infrared coagulation or laser coagulation.

Soiling is an unpleasant symptom caused by prolapse (or outpouching) of the membrane that lines the lower rectum through the anus. As the membrane protrudes out, solid or liquid stool transfers to the undergarments. Hemorrhoid banding, as described earlier, is remarkably effective for this problem. The healing of the area that's been banded is accompanied by scar tissue that attaches the membrane to the underlying muscle, and this attachment reduces the ability of the membrane to prolapse.

Hemorrhoids can be excised (cut out) by a colorectal surgeon. Surgery may be necessary for severe pain that does not respond to conservative measures or cannot be treated by incision and clot removal. Additional indications for hemorrhoid surgery include large or bothersome hemorrhoids (especially external) and bleeding or painful hemorrhoids that do not respond to minimally invasive procedures. Pain after hemorrhoid surgery can be significant but can be managed by the colorectal surgeon.

Anal itching can be a result of a yeast infection, excessive wiping, or skin tags that are difficult to clean. Sitz baths can be helpful, and over-the-counter creams are available for yeast infections. Itching from other causes may respond to hydrocortisone cream, but this medication should not be used for more than a few weeks.

Anal fissure can cause acute or chronic anal pain, which is often severe, especially after a bowel movement. The fissure is a thin, hairline tear in the anal lining caused by trauma such as hard stool, vaginal delivery, or anal sex. Recurrences are common. Initial treatment is with sitz baths, stool softeners, dietary fiber, and nitroglycerin ointment. For chronic anal fissure that does not respond to initial treatment, injections of botulinum toxin (Botox) or surgical repair is considered.

TAKE-HOME MESSAGES

- Hemorrhoids are normal veins in the anal canal. They usually do not cause symptoms but can be associated with pain, bleeding, or itching.
- Initial treatment of hemorrhoids is with fiber, stool softeners, oral fluids, and sitz baths.
- Prescription medications such as nitroglycerin ointment or hydrocortisone can be very effective.
- Sudden, severe anorectal pain with a new bulge may be a thrombosed hemorrhoid. If this occurs, call your doctor immediately; a small incision can be made in the hemorrhoid and the clot removed, but this must be done within forty-eight hours of the onset of symptoms.
- Minimally invasive procedures such as hemorrhoid banding can reduce or eliminate bleeding, pain, or soiling. The most definitive procedure is surgical removal.

13

Evaluation of the Esophagus, Stomach, and Small Intestine

The upper GI tract is generally examined because of certain symptoms or abnormal test results. Those symptoms include heartburn, trouble swallowing, abdominal pain, nausea, vomiting, and bleeding. Other reasons for evaluating the upper GI tract are anemia, laboratory tests suggestive of celiac disease, follow-up of ulcers after treatment, food becoming stuck in the esophagus, or foreign body ingestion.

GI bleeding may be evident by obvious blood in the stool or black stool. Black stool (or melena) most commonly denotes an upper GI source, such as bleeding from ulcers in the esophagus, stomach, or duodenum. Red blood in the stool, in contrast, suggests lower GI bleeding, which could result from diverticulosis, colon cancer, or hemorrhoids. There are many exceptions to this, however, and in many instances of GI bleeding, the stools may be burgundy, maroon, or some other hue that is intermediate between black and red. A proper evaluation of GI bleeding usually requires both upper and lower GI assessments. GI bleeding can result from aspirin (even low dose) and ibuprofen, naproxen, and similar medications. These drugs, collectively known as non-steroidal anti-inflammatory drugs (NSAIDs), can cause erosions or ulcers in any part of the digestive tract, but most commonly in the stomach or small intestine.

The common endoscopic procedure for the upper GI tract is called an **esophagogastroduodenoscopy (EGD),** also called an **upper GI endoscopy**. It involves the use of a flexible scope which is shorter and thinner than the colonoscope. The upper GI tract can also be studied by various imaging procedures, including the upper GI series, in which barium is swallowed and X-rays are taken, and a CT scan (see glossary). The bile and pancreatic ducts can be evaluated by a procedure known as endoscopic retrograde chol-

---

MORE ON MELENA

- Melena is a black stool with a tarry consistency and a strong, unmistakable odor.
- Melena indicates bleeding, usually from the upper GI tract.
- After bleeding into the upper GI tract, the blood travels downstream and becomes partially digested, leading to the black color.
- Taking iron by mouth, as well as Pepto-Bismol or charcoal tablets, can cause dark or even black stools, but in these cases the stool does not have an abnormal odor. Normal stool color will return when these agents are stopped.
- Upper GI bleeding can be serious or even life-threatening. Melena, especially with dizziness, light-headedness, or passing out, is a medical emergency and warrants an immediate trip to the nearest emergency facility.

---

angiopancreatography (ERCP) in which a special type of upper scope called a duodenoscope is used (see section below on cleaning and disinfection, and chapter 16, "Gallbladder and Pancreas"). The EGD provides the advantage of directly viewing the inner lining of the esophagus, stomach, and first part of the small intestine. It also allows the endoscopist to take biopsies and perform other interventions discussed later in this chapter. As with a colonoscopy, very clear images can be seen via EGD (as seen in figure 13.1).

Whether or not you have an EGD is up to you and your primary physician or gastroenterologist. Chapter 15, "Disorders of the Stomach and Small Intestine, Including Celiac Disease," reviews many of the conditions that can be diagnosed and treated using this procedure.

No laxatives are needed to prepare for an EGD. It's very important, however, that your stomach is empty before the procedure. You should have no solid food after midnight (unlike colonoscopy, where you have only clear liquids the day before) and no liquids for at least six hours before your procedure. As with colonoscopy, critical medications (for heart, blood pressure, or seizure problems) may be taken in the morning with a small sip of water, but please confirm this with your gastroenterologist. If there is residual food or fluid in the stomach, there is an increased risk of aspiration, i.e., inhalation of the stomach contents into the lungs. Because aspiration can lead to a serious pneumonia, your procedure may be canceled if you do not follow the instructions regarding nothing by mouth. EGD procedures are frequently canceled because the patient failed to remember not to eat or drink in the morning. Depending on the type and amount of food or drink consumed and the elapsed time since such consumption, it may be possible to wait and do the EGD a few hours later.

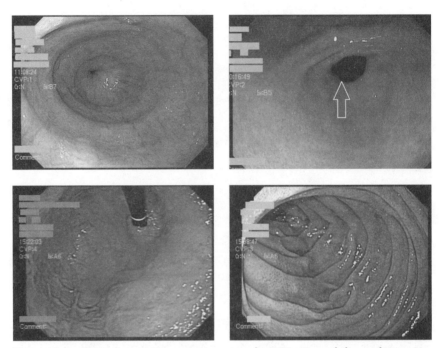

Figure 13.1. Normal upper GI anatomy as seen by EGD. Upper left: esophagus. Upper right: lower stomach, or antrum. Arrow: pylorus. Lower left: upper stomach. Lower right: duodenum (part of small intestine).

Source: David M. Novick, *Esophagus,* July 2016.

If you did follow all instructions and nevertheless have food in the stomach, you may have gastroparesis, a condition in which the stomach does not empty properly.

Your pre-procedure evaluation will be similar to that for a colonoscopy. Either conscious sedation or TIVA may be used. It's possible to do an EGD with no sedation, but this is very rarely done. Before the scope is inserted, a plastic bite block is placed in the mouth in order to prevent you from biting the scope and to protect your teeth. The scope is passed over the tongue into the pharynx (back of throat) and then into the esophagus (food pipe). It does not go into the trachea (windpipe). After reaching the esophagus, the scope is gradually advanced into the stomach and the duodenum (the first part of the small intestine).

Many interventions are possible during an EGD. Biopsies (tissue samples) can be taken from the esophagus, stomach, or duodenum in a similar fashion to those done at colonoscopy (see chapter 3, "The Colonoscopy"). Biopsies are performed not only to exclude cancer but also to evaluate various types of inflammation, to detect a stomach bacteria called *Helicobacter pylori* that can cause ulcers or cancer, or to diagnose celiac disease. A stricture (narrowing) of the esophagus can be dilated (stretched open) using a balloon or a thick rubber tube. Polyps can be removed using the same methods as for colonoscopy. A bleeding site, usually an ulcer, can be controlled with several methods. It can be injected with a drug that constricts blood vessels, cauterized with the heater probe, and/or closed up with a clip. These interventions are very effective in stopping bleeding, and surgery is rarely needed.

Dilated veins in the esophagus, known as varices and seen in patients with cirrhosis of the liver, can be pinched off by placing a rubber band around them. See chapter 18, "Cirrhosis and the Spectrum of Liver Disease," for more discussion on varices. This procedure, known as variceal ligation, is only done at the hospital because of the risk of bleeding during the procedure and the possible need for more intense anesthesia services than those provided in an outpatient center.

EGD is exceptionally safe. Complications are extremely rare and are much less common than with colonoscopy. Perforation of the esophagus can occur after dilation of the esophagus with any method, and this complication requires admission to the hospital. Surgery is sometimes required. Esophageal perforation is suggested by significant chest pain following dilation. Bleeding can occur, especially after the interventions discussed earlier. Aspiration of stomach contents into the lungs is also very rare but more common than with colonoscopy. Most complications can be managed effectively, especially if they are recognized early.

Recovery after EGD is similar to that for colonoscopy (see chapter 4, "Recovery after Colonoscopy"). You should have no plans for the remainder of the day after your EGD, other than to relax at home. If you have been sedated, you may not drive, sign any documents, or operate any equipment that requires alertness.

CLEANING AND DISINFECTION OF ENDOSCOPES

Endoscopes for GI tract evaluation, including those for EGD, ERCP, and colonoscopy, come in contact with fluids and tissues containing a wide range of microorganisms. These scopes are thoroughly cleaned and disinfected between each use. Effective procedures to accomplish this have been developed by the GI societies and must be carefully followed.

Very rarely, bacterial infections or hepatitis B or C virus infections have been transmitted by contaminated endoscopes.[1] Such cases are considered to have been due to failure to follow standard disinfection or infection control procedures.[2]

WHAT HAPPENED TO JOAN RIVERS?

Comedian Joan Rivers died on September 4, 2014, several days after she had a laryngoscopy* and an EGD with propofol anesthesia in an outpatient endoscopy center. She underwent these procedures to address voice changes and symptoms of reflux. The medical examiner reported that she died of a respiratory arrest (stopped breathing) that led to the type of brain injury associated with insufficient oxygen supply. The reason that she stopped breathing was not stated. The report also added that respiratory arrest is a known complication of anesthesia and of these procedures.[3–5]

News reports[6,7] mentioned allegations of unprofessional and possibly negligent actions or omissions during Ms. Rivers's procedure, including the following:

- Ms. Rivers's personal ear, nose, and throat (ENT) physician was present and may have participated in the procedure despite not having been credentialed at that center.
- A vocal cord biopsy was done, and it caused swelling or spasm of Ms. Rivers's vocal cords leading to blockage of her airway and inability to breathe. The endoscopy center in question does not normally do vocal cord biopsies, and many authorities consider vocal cord biopsy to be a hospital procedure.
- In similar emergency situations, the anesthesiologist can make an incision into the trachea (windpipe), bypassing the vocal cord obstruction and allowing air to enter the lungs.
- There were delays in starting cardiopulmonary resuscitation (CPR) and in calling 911.

Although a small number of complications is inevitable for any type of procedure, complications are more likely to occur when exceptions are made to standard operating procedure, even (and sometimes especially) when requested by the patient. Adhering to established protocols and safety assessments such as "time out" (see chapter 2, "Sedation and Anesthesia") will reduce the number of complications in any facility. As others have noted,[8] celebrities or influential people may receive worse care because exceptions are made for them.

*An endoscopic procedure performed by ENT physicians in which a very thin scope is used to view the larynx (voice box).

In 2013, an outbreak of infection with carbapenem-resistant Enterobacteriaceae (CRE), a group of bacteria resistant to most antibiotics and referred to in the lay press as "superbugs," was identified and linked to the use of duodenoscopes.[9] In this outbreak, and others that followed, proper cleaning and disinfection procedures were followed. This suggests that the greater complexity of the side-viewing duodenoscopes used for ERCP is an important factor. Duodenoscopes have a separate channel (elevator) which orients the various devices used for biliary and pancreatic interventions and is difficult to completely clean and disinfect.[10] In a recent study, the greatest risk of CRE transmission was in patients who were hospitalized, had a biliary stent placed, or who had cholangiocarcinoma.[11]

More meticulous cleaning of duodenoscopes, redesign of the elevator, checking the scopes for bacterial growth before reuse, and changing the standard cleaning procedure from high-level disinfection to gas sterilization are being studied in order to prevent future transmission of CRE by duodenoscopes. ERCP remains the safest and least invasive approach for many serious diseases of the pancreas and biliary tract.[12]

THE SMALL INTESTINE

Most of the small intestine is inaccessible to the scopes used for EGD and even the longer scope used for colonoscopy. When the small bowel needs to be investigated, one option is to insert a (thoroughly cleaned) pediatric colonoscope through the mouth. This scope can be advanced farther into the small intestine than the scope used for an EGD but will still leave two-thirds or more of the small intestine unseen. Even longer scopes exist but are less readily available and have limitations of their own. They may coil excessively in the stomach, limiting the distance reached. This can be overcome by use of an overtube, a stiff, hollow single-use tube that fits over the last two feet of the scope. The overtube stays in the stomach and keeps the scope from coiling. The small-bowel scope, or enteroscope, is passed through the overtube and then through the outlet of the stomach into the small intestine. Use of an overtube slightly increases the risk of the procedure. Also, the success rate of the enteroscope is increased with the use of a fluoroscope, which allows visualization of the scope within the body by live X-ray images on a fluorescent screen. However, fluoroscopy contributes radiation exposure, which can be significant if not done carefully.

In 2001, a disposable wireless capsule the size of a large pill was approved for small-bowel imaging. The capsule contains light-emitting diodes (LEDs) and a camera, lens, battery, transmitter, and antenna. It takes two pictures per second and beams the images to a receiver that the patient wears around his or her waist. The capsule does not need to be retrieved after it is passed out in the stool. The receiver is turned in after eight hours, and the images are uploaded to a computer for viewing by the doctor. Figure 13.2 shows the small-bowel capsule.

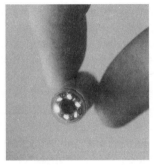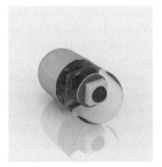

Figure 13.2.   Once ingested, the endoscopic video capsule, equipped with a camera, allows the complete exploration of the small intestine.
Source: Phanie/Alamy (left); Cosinart/Thinkstock photos (right).

If you have a capsule endoscopy, you will be advised to check your stools for the capsule so that your doctor knows that it has passed completely through you. If it is not seen by two weeks, a simple X-ray will ensure that the capsule has passed and is not stuck in you. It's rare that the capsule does not pass, that is, it gets stuck. This generally causes no immediate problem and can be helpful in diagnosing various types of bowel narrowing or obstruction. A small operation is needed to remove a capsule that is stuck. Capsule endoscopy is very helpful when someone has gastrointestinal bleeding, and EGD and colonoscopy fail to reveal the source.

TAKE-HOME MESSAGES

- GI bleeding can result from aspirin (even low dose) and ibuprofen, naproxen, and similar medications. These may cause ulcers of the stomach or small intestine. Use them with caution, under your doctor's supervision.
- An EGD is used to evaluate many GI complaints, including heartburn, trouble swallowing, abdominal pain, nausea, vomiting, and bleeding.
- Black stools with a tarry consistency (melena) usually indicate bleeding, most commonly in the upper GI tract. Blood gets partially digested as it goes downstream, leading to the black color. Such bleeding can be serious. Melena, especially with dizziness, warrants an immediate trip to the nearest emergency room.
- Bleeding encountered during an EGD can be stopped using an injection of epinephrine to constrict blood vessels, heater probe cautery, a clip, or a combination of these. Surgery is rarely needed.
- Foreign bodies lodged in the esophagus can be removed via an EGD.

- If you swallow something and have severe pain, or if food gets stuck such that you cannot swallow your own saliva, go to the nearest ER for evaluation for an emergency EGD.
- To reduce the risk of aspiration or accidental swallowing of foreign objects, do not talk when actively chewing, and do not use your mouth to hold objects.
- The risk of contracting an infection from a contaminated endoscope, while not zero, is extremely minimal.

14

Heartburn and Reflux

Heartburn affects sixty million Americans, and about fifteen million have it every day.[1] Heartburn is commonly described as a burning pain in the mid-chest. It can extend up to the throat or down to the abdomen. It is strongly associated with gastroesophageal reflux (GE reflux), which is the movement of stomach contents into the esophagus. Here is some other reflux terminology:

- **Gastroesophageal reflux disease (GERD):** A general term for the symptoms and manifestations of GE reflux.
- **Acid reflux:** Often used synonymously with GE reflux, but reflux can be acidic or nonacidic.
- **Reflux esophagitis:** The finding of inflammation of the esophagus on biopsy obtained during an EGD.
- **Hiatus hernia:** The slippage of a portion of the stomach up through the diaphragm and into the chest. Often associated with reflux, but one can have reflux without hiatus hernia, and hiatus hernia without reflux.
- **Lower esophageal sphincter:** The muscles in the lowest, or most distal, part of the esophagus that are normally contracted to prevent stomach contents from refluxing into the esophagus. This sphincter does not function optimally in patients with GERD. During swallowing, the muscles of the lower esophageal sphincter relax to let the food go down from the esophagus into the stomach.

This chapter will cover GERD, some conditions with similar symptoms, and complications of GERD including stricture of the esophagus, Barrett's esophagus, and esophageal cancer.

HEARTBURN OR HEART ATTACK?

Both can cause chest pain, but a heart attack is a true emergency and requires immediate medical attention. Go to the nearest emergency room immediately if your chest pain has ANY of the following symptoms:

- Starts suddenly
- Doesn't go away
- Gets worse
- Is accompanied by dizziness, shortness of breath, sweating, nausea, or palpitations (feeling your heart beating)
- Gets worse with exertion

While most chest pain is not related to heart problems (in fact, GE reflux is a more common cause) it's better to be safe than sorry. Heart attacks can be fatal.

There is an old saying in medicine that "patients don't follow the textbook." This means that some patients do not have typical or classical symptoms, and they may come to medical attention for complaints that do not immediately suggest the underlying diagnosis. Accordingly, there are other symptoms of GERD besides heartburn, including cough, hoarseness, frequent throat clearing, and asthma. GE reflux may trigger asthma when tiny acid particles enter the lungs after having come up from the stomach into the throat, a process known as aspiration. GERD is sometimes diagnosed by ear, nose, and throat (ENT) physicians, either because of some of the above symptoms or with abnormal findings at laryngoscopy (examination of the larynx, or voice box), though such findings must be confirmed by additional testing.

ALARM SYMPTOMS

Prompt evaluation of heartburn or reflux, usually including an EGD, is recommended if any of the following are present:

- Trouble or pain on swallowing
- Weight loss
- Vomiting
- Vomiting blood or passing black or maroon-colored stools
- Anemia

NON-MEDICAL HEARTBURN TREATMENTS

There are several non-medical measures that can help with heartburn:

- Do not eat late at night. Do not eat or drink anything for three to four hours before going to sleep. If your mouth gets dry, take ice chips. Evening medications may be taken with a small amount of water, and you should wait a few minutes after taking them before lying down.
- Do not lie down after eating. When you lie down, stomach contents can more easily reflux into the chest. It's better to be upright after eating— take a walk or do the dishes!
- Avoid very large meals.
- Avoid foods that predictably cause you to have heartburn. Tomato products, citrus fruits, chocolate, and mints are common offenders. If you tolerate these foods, you may take them in moderation.
- Raise the head of the bed four to six inches. Use wood blocks, old phonebooks, or bed blocks purchased at home-furnishing stores.
- Reduce or eliminate caffeine, carbonated beverages, and alcohol.
- Quit smoking. Discontinue other tobacco products.
- Lose weight (see chapter 19, "Healthy Eating").

MEDICATIONS FOR HEARTBURN

Medications are often needed to control heartburn and to treat the complications of GERD. The most common group of drugs in use today are the proton pump inhibitors (PPIs), most of which are available as generic drugs, that is, they are no longer patent protected and can be made by competing companies. Most PPIs are available over the counter, without a doctor's prescription, for a fourteen-day course. PPIs block most or all acid produced by the stomach and are very effective for heartburn. Your doctor may recommend a trial of a PPI for six to eight weeks to confirm the diagnosis of GERD, and a positive response may make further testing unnecessary. Most PPIs work better when taken on an empty stomach, thirty to sixty minutes before a meal. Some people take them at bedtime, but they are much less effective when taken at that time. For nighttime use, the older acid blockers (known as H2 blockers) such as ranitidine (Zantac) or famotidine (Pepcid) are preferred.

The commonly prescribed PPIs are:

- Omeprazole (Prilosec)
- Omeprazole/sodium bicarbonate (Zegerid)

- Lansoprazole (Prevacid)
- Dexlansoprazole (DEXILANT)
- Rabeprazole sodium (ACEIPHEX)
- Pantoprazole sodium (PROTONIX)
- Esomeprazole (Nexium)

A challenging area of medical management is *how long to continue PPIs*. Many people find that their heartburn comes back as soon as they stop their PPI and therefore take PPIs indefinitely. Although PPIs are safe for long-term use, there are some notes of caution (discussed later), and it is desirable to discontinue them if possible after several months. Taking PPIs every other day, dose reduction, and transitioning to H2 blockers may be useful strategies. In general, it is much easier to start PPIs (and many other medications) than to stop them; **it is a good idea to periodically review your medications with your doctor**. Patients with ulcers in the esophagus, strictures, or Barrett's esophagus will often require long-term PPI treatment.

For decades, PPIs have been considered to be very safe. In recent years, a number of concerns have been raised about possible or actual adverse effects of these medications. These are:

- Reduced bone density
- Increased risk of fractures
- Reduced magnesium level
- Reduced B12 level
- Increased risk of *Clostridium difficile* infection
- Increased risk of pneumonia
- Drug interactions
- Increased risk of acute kidney injury
- Increased risk of chronic kidney disease
- Increased risk of dementia

A significant concern about PPI treatment is its impact on calcium and bone health. PPIs reduce the absorption of calcium from the GI tract, and this may lead to reduced bone density and an increased risk of fractures. The risk is greater in elderly people and those taking PPIs twice daily.[2] The best way to prevent this is with increased calcium in the diet. The following foods are rich in calcium:

- Milk and other dairy products
- Fortified orange juice (however, many patients with GERD cannot tolerate this)

- Deep green vegetables, e.g., kale, broccoli, spinach, collard greens, watercress, bok choy
- Salmon and sardines (the best being canned products that contain bones)
- Some fortified breakfast cereals (check label)
- Miscellaneous: white beans, almonds, figs, dates, soy, sesame or sunflower seeds, blackstrap molasses

Calcium supplements are another option. If used, take at least twice daily and no more than 500 mg at one time. Calcium citrate may be better absorbed by people on PPIs than calcium carbonate. There have been some reports linking calcium supplements and cardiac events. The issue is not settled at this time, hence the advice to get calcium through food if possible. PPIs can also reduce the absorption of magnesium and vitamin B12. The low magnesium does not always improve with magnesium supplements and sometimes does not resolve unless PPIs are discontinued.[3]

VITAMIN D

A surprising number of people are deficient in vitamin D, which helps deposit calcium into bone. Ask your doctor to check your level, especially if you are taking PPIs.

PPIs can also increase the risk of certain infections, especially *C. difficile* (or C-diff). Gastric acid is one of the many barriers to infection and is partially or completely blocked by the PPI. In the case of C-diff, acid defends against the spores (inactive forms of the bacteria, like tiny seeds) by which C-diff is spread. Also, PPIs may interact with certain medications, notably the combination of ledipasvir and sofosbuvir (HARVONI), a very effective treatment for some strains of hepatitis C. Taking a low dose of a PPI at the same time as Harvoni is usually acceptable. Discuss all drug interaction questions with your physician. See chapter 11, *"Clostridium difficile* Infection, or C-diff," for more information on C-diff.

In an article published online in January 2016 and subsequently in print, a study of two large groups of patients showed an association of PPIs with chronic kidney disease.[4] PPI users were more likely to have chronic kidney disease than those who did not use PPIs and also than those who used H2 blockers. The association with PPI and chronic kidney disease was strengthened by the observation that twice daily PPI users had a significantly higher risk of chronic kidney disease when compared with those using PPI once per day. This study also confirmed the previously reported[5] association of PPI use with acute kidney injury. PPIs could cause chronic kidney disease through their association with low magnesium levels, a risk factor for kidney disease, or by repeated episodes of acute kidney injury.[6]

This type of study reports observations but cannot prove causation, i.e., that PPI use causes chronic kidney disease. There may be other risk factors that are associated with both PPI use and chronic kidney disease that were not measured or are not known. Further research is needed to determine whether PPIs cause chronic kidney disease.

One month after the online publication of the study on chronic kidney disease, an article was published online linking PPIs with dementia.[7] The research was based on data from insurance claims from 73,679 patients age seventy-five or older. The analysis took into account some but not all of the factors that could contribute to dementia; it controlled for age, sex, use of five or more medications other than PPIs, and the diagnoses of stroke, depression, coronary artery (heart) disease, and diabetes. The study did not differentiate between various types of dementia. The authors make reference to a previous, more intensive but much smaller study done by the same group of investigators, which revealed an increased risk of dementia in people taking PPIs.[8] In the present study, the researchers found that the patients receiving PPIs were more likely to have a diagnosis of dementia than those not taking PPIs.

This study must be taken seriously, but there are several reservations. First, like the study on chronic kidney disease, the presence of a statistical association does not prove that PPIs cause dementia. Second, there could be other known or unknown factors that increase the risk of both PPI use and dementia that were not assessed in this study. Some possible examples are differences in educational level, diet, smoking, alcohol use, and obesity. There is a very strong inverse relationship between the risk of dementia and educational level[9] (with the inverse relationship, low educational level is associated with a high risk of dementia). The role of these factors needs to be assessed in future studies. Third, diagnoses made on insurance claims may not be as precise as those determined by researchers. The authors state that additional research is necessary in order to establish a causal relationship between PPIs and dementia.[10]

While we do not know whether PPIs cause chronic kidney disease or dementia, it is important to keep in mind that PPIs are probably not as safe as previously thought. Physicians and patients need to be more careful about the use of PPIs, which are among the most commonly prescribed medications today. There is evidence that PPIs are overprescribed.[11] Prescriptions for PPIs are frequently continued long after the condition for which they were prescribed has resolved. Some patients, such as those with Barrett's esophagus, GERD that will not respond to any other treatment, GI symptoms from nonsteroidal anti-inflammatory drugs (NSAIDs) that are needed for other conditions, and ulcers of unknown cause that continue to recur, may require long-term PPI treatment. All PPI prescriptions and over-the-counter use should be reevaluated periodically and discontinued when possible.

The main alternatives to PPIs are the H2 blockers (ranitidine, famotidine, and others) and antacids. In some patients, reflux may be controlled using H2 blockers twice daily. H2 blockers work more quickly than PPIs but are less potent. They are often useful for nighttime reflux, though this benefit may diminish with time. H2 blockers may be useful when someone stops their PPI and develops increased heartburn or reflux. Antacids containing aluminum, magnesium, or calcium are useful for immediate but short-term symptom relief.

"MY HEARTBURN TREATMENT ISN'T WORKING!"

It may not be heartburn. Heart disease and other conditions may have similar symptoms. Discuss evaluation for other causes with your primary care physician.

TESTING

As noted earlier, a trial of PPI can help to establish the diagnosis of GERD. EGD is recommended for patients with alarm symptoms, non-responders to PPIs, and those in whom the diagnosis is uncertain. An EGD is also done when there are risk factors for Barrett's esophagus (discussed later in this chapter), to follow up on esophageal ulcers or severe inflammation to ensure healing, or to dilate strictures or rings in people with trouble swallowing.

When the diagnosis is still unclear after PPI trial and endoscopy, pH monitoring can be useful (pH is a unit of acidity). A probe is placed in the lower esophagus by the scope, and it beams the data to a receiver that the patient wears. Other technologies also exist for pH measurement. This test can confirm that acid is refluxing into the esophagus. It can also help determine if asthma is reflux related.

OVERLAPPING GI CONDITIONS

There are many gastrointestinal problems with similar symptoms to GERD. Two of them are **pill esophagitis** and **eosinophilic esophagitis**. Pill esophagitis is an erosion or ulcer that occurs from a pill being swallowed with little or no water. Pain or bleeding may result. Pill esophagitis is more common in young people or those in a hurry. It's best to drink a generous amount of water when swallowing pills, unless you have GERD and must take medications at bedtime. In this case, take just enough to get the pill down.

Eosinophilic esophagitis is an inflammation of the esophagus characterized by infiltration by large numbers of eosinophils (a type of white blood cell that is commonly seen in allergic reactions). It's closely associated with asthma, food allergy, and other allergic conditions. Rare before 1990, it has become one of the most common causes of trouble swallowing in teenagers and young adults.[12] Symptoms include trouble swallowing, reflux-like symptoms, and food impaction (food stuck in esophagus). Eosinophilic esophagitis may be responsible for up to 54 percent of food impactions.[13] It is most common in young adult males. The EGD shows a pattern of multiple ridges, stacked rings, or strictures, and biopsy shows many eosinophils. There's an increased risk of perforation of the esophagus following EGD with dilation in patients with eosinophilic esophagitis. Treatment includes the use of a PPI or a corticosteroid inhaler (as used for asthma, but the mist from the inhaler is swallowed, not inhaled). Allergy testing is recommended for non-responders.

SURGERY FOR GERD

Surgery is an option for patients who do not wish to take PPIs long term, do not comply with therapy, or who do not respond well to treatment despite documented GERD. The most common surgical procedure is a Nissen fundoplication, in which the fundus of the stomach (the upper, dome-like part of the stomach) is wrapped around the junction of the esophagus and stomach, thereby tightening the opening and reducing reflux. In other words, the Nissen procedure compensates for the failure of the lower esophageal sphincter to remain contracted and prevent reflux. The procedure can be done laparoscopically, and about 85–90 percent of patients have improvement in symptoms. Post-operative complications include trouble swallowing (often requiring dilation) and bloating. Also, many patients who have anti-reflux surgery end up back on PPI despite initial good results.

ESOPHAGEAL ULCER

An ulcer is a disruption of the membrane lining any part of the GI tract. Ulcers are often painful but may have no symptoms. They can be superficial or can form a crater, which in turn can erode into a blood vessel, causing bleeding. A very deep ulcer can lead to perforation. Ulcers in the GI tract can be caused by unopposed acid, by aspirin or NSAIDs; e.g., ibuprofen, naproxen, or by a bacteria called *Helicobacter pylori,* located in the stomach or duodenum (see chapter 15, "Disorders of the Stomach and Small Intestine, Including Celiac Disease"). Ulcers in the upper GI tract are commonly diagnosed by EGD. Ulcers of the esophagus are commonly seen with untreated reflux or reflux that is non-responsive to PPI. Common approaches to treatment include the following:

- Start a PPI (if the patient is not already on one).
- Change the dose, increase to twice daily, or change to a different PPI (if the patient is already on one).
- Add an H2 blocker.
- Add sucralfate, a medication that adheres to the surface of the ulcer and protects it against acid, pepsin, or bile salts (see glossary).
- Encourage the non-medical approaches to reflux mentioned earlier.

A follow-up EGD in eight weeks is recommended to ensure that the ulcers are healing. A non-healing ulcer should be biopsied to exclude cancer. Also, Barrett's esophagus is often apparent after the healing of an esophageal ulcer, and biopsies are needed in this situation as well.

ESOPHAGEAL STRICTURES AND RINGS

Recurrent GE reflux may lead to inflammation in the lower esophagus, and this inflammation may heal with the formation of scar tissue. With repetition of this process over many years, the scar tissue can become sufficient to narrow the lumen (opening of the inside of the esophagus), forming a stricture. Strictures lead to trouble swallowing, painful swallowing, and food impaction. They are often associated with inflammation or ulcers of the esophagus.

Treatment includes dilation, during which the narrowed segment of the esophagus is gently widened (dilated). Dilation can be done using a balloon which is passed through the scope while deflated, and then inflated in the lumen of the esophagus in the vicinity of the stricture. It is deflated and removed afterward (see figure 14.1).

Alternative methods for dilation involve the passage of a tapered rubber tube called a bougie through the esophagus. Sometimes a thin wire is passed through the scope and then the scope is withdrawn, leaving the guide wire in place; the dilator is then passed over the guide wire to ensure proper place-

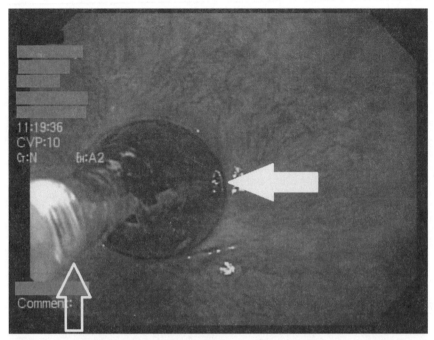

11:19:36
CVP:10
Gr:N   Br:A2

Commen :

Figure 14.1. A balloon at the end of a catheter has been passed through the scope and is then inflated in the lumen of the esophagus at an area of narrowing. Open arrow: catheter. Closed arrow: balloon.
Source: David M. Novick, *Balloon Dilation,* July 2016.

ment. Most patients with strictures have a good response to dilation by any of these methods. Once a patient has had a dilation for a stricture, it's likely that he or she will need it again at some point. Very rarely, esophageal dilation can cause perforation of the esophagus, for which urgent surgical repair is required. Stricture patients are usually managed on PPI medications in an attempt to prevent further inflammation resulting from reflux.

Esophageal rings are smooth, thin structures that encircle the lumen of the esophagus. When they appear at the gastroesophageal junction, they are known as Schatzki rings. While the relationship of esophageal rings to reflux is unclear, they can definitely cause trouble swallowing solid food. Rings are treated with dilation when symptoms are present.

BARRETT'S ESOPHAGUS

Barrett's esophagus is a consequence of longstanding GE reflux, with or without symptoms. It is common: approximately 5.6 percent of adults in the

United States have Barrett's esophagus.[14] It is important because it predisposes to cancer. **Barrett's esophagus can occur in people with no symptoms of reflux**. It has several key features:

- An irregular border between the esophagus and stomach, in which the membrane from the stomach appears to project up into the esophagus (see figure 14.2).
- Cells in the area of Barrett's that resemble small intestine rather than esophagus or stomach (known as intestinal metaplasia). Diagnosis is made by biopsy.
- A small but definite association of Barrett's esophagus with a particular type of cancer of the esophagus called adenocarcinoma.

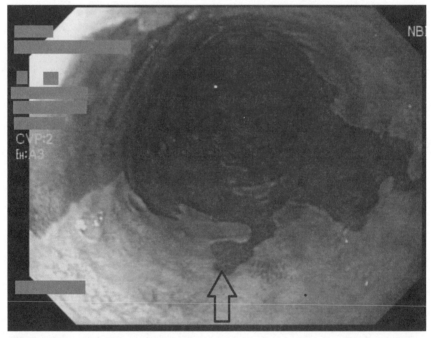

Figure 14.2. Barrett's esophagus. The arrow shows an irregular border between normal-appearing esophagus and a portion of lower esophagus replaced by cells that resemble those of the intestine (darker area).

Source: David M. Novick, *Barrett's Esophagus*, July 2016.

The most important risk factors for Barrett's esophagus and esophageal adenocarcinoma are identical.[15] They include the following:

- Age fifty or older
- White males
- Obesity (especially intra-abdominal)
- Smoking
- Longstanding heartburn

Other risk factors are a family history of GERD and eating lots of processed food or red meat. **If you have GERD plus one or more of these risk factors, discuss a screening EGD with your doctor**. The greater the number of risk factors, the higher the risk. A man with GERD over age fifty who is obese and a smoker will have a substantial risk of Barrett's esophagus.[16] Barrett's esophagus is less common in African Americans, and a diet high in fruits and vegetables is associated with reduced risk of Barrett's esophagus and esophageal carcinoma. The regular use of aspirin or NSAIDs is also associated with a reduced risk of both conditions, but is not recommended as the sole treatment.

The surveillance of Barrett's esophagus consists of a follow-up EGD with multiple biopsies within one year and then every three years. The most important factor is either the presence or absence of dysplasia (an abnormal size, shape, or arrangement of the cells that normally is a forerunner of cancer). Dysplasia can be low or high grade; high-grade dysplasia is characterized by more severe changes and greater variability in the cells. Both types of dysplasia can progress to cancer, with more rapid progression in high-grade dysplasia. Diagnosing dysplasia on biopsies can be challenging, and biopsy slides should be reviewed by one or more expert pathologists.

Unlike the situation with colon cancer, screening of reflux patients with EGD has not had an impact on the rate of esophageal adenocarcinoma. Patients with esophageal adenocarcinoma often have no GE reflux. A better way to identify Barrett's esophagus and the subgroup most likely to develop cancer is urgently needed. Until this is accomplished, an EGD remains the best approach for screening.

Dysplasia in a patient with Barrett's esophagus requires definitive treatment. Two new techniques can be used to treat Barrett's esophagus with dysplasia, and they can be done by a gastroenterologist during an EGD, greatly reducing the need for surgery:

- **Radiofrequency ablation**: a special balloon delivers multiple pulses of intense heat energy to the inner lining of the esophagus in the affected area, sparing deeper tissue.

  ✓ Definitely recommended for high-grade dysplasia in Barrett's esophagus; many authorities advise it for low-grade dysplasia as well.

  ✓ Eighty percent response rate, with several follow-up procedures required.

- **Endoscopic mucosal resection**: a complete removal of the involved parts of the inner lining of the esophagus via an endoscope. This is used for visible nodules or superficial adenocarcinoma.

  ✓ Usually done along with radiofrequency ablation

Both procedures must be done by a physician experienced in these techniques. Complications of these procedures include chest pain, bleeding, stricture, and perforation.

It's standard practice to treat patients with Barrett's esophagus and GERD with PPIs for an indefinite duration due to the possibility that doing so will prevent cancer, although the evidence for this is modest. It's controversial whether patients with Barrett's esophagus without symptoms of GE reflux should be similarly treated.

ESOPHAGEAL CANCER

There are two types of esophageal cancer: **adenocarcinoma** and **squamous cell carcinoma**. Although adenocarcinoma is more common in the United States and Europe, and continues to rise in incidence, squamous cell carcinoma is the most common type worldwide. Squamous cell carcinoma is equally common in men and women and is most common in the upper or mid-esophagus, whereas adenocarcinoma is much more common in men and is found mainly in the lower (distal) esophagus. In 2016, 16,910 new cases of esophageal cancer and 15,690 deaths were expected in the United States.[17]

The incidence of adenocarcinoma of the esophagus in the United States has progressively increased from 3.6 cases per million in 1973 to 25.6 per million in 2006, although the annual *rate* of increase slowed from 8.2 percent before 1996 to 1.3 percent subsequently.[18] In contrast, squamous cell carcinoma has declined in incidence.

In one study, a majority of esophageal adenocarcinomas were attributable to smoking, being overweight, reflux symptoms, and low fruit and vegetable consumption.[19]

Both types of cancer have symptoms that include trouble swallowing, weight loss, anemia, or poorly controlled reflux. Either type may also have no symptoms and may be diagnosed unexpectedly during an EGD or an imaging procedure. If esophageal cancer is found, the next step is a visit with an oncologist, followed by staging. The following box shows a simplified version of staging of esophageal cancer.[20]

STAGING OF ESOPHAGEAL CANCER

Stage 0: The tumor remains within the inner membrane (mucosa) lining the esophagus.

Stage I: The tumor invades through the mucosa but has not reached the muscle layer of the esophagus. No involvement of lymph nodes or distant sites.

Stage II: The tumor invades the muscle layer of the esophagus. Lymph nodes may or may not be involved.

Stage III: The tumor invades through the muscle layer of the esophagus and involves lymph nodes or other areas adjacent to the esophagus.

Stage IV: The tumor has metastasized to distant lymph nodes or organs.

Staging is done at a multidisciplinary conference using information from the EGD and CT scans. Two other tests have increased the accuracy of the staging of esophageal cancer:

- Endoscopic ultrasound
- Positron emission tomography (PET) scan

Endoscopic ultrasound is an ultrasound done inside the body using a scope that resembles the scope used for EGD but has an ultrasound probe on the tip. This instrument allows a more accurate assessment of the depth of invasion of these tumors, as well as the involvement of adjacent lymph nodes. Using a very thin needle that is passed through the scope and into the area of interest (fine-needle aspiration), cells from the tumor or lymph nodes can be withdrawn by the gastroenterologist.

PET scanning can identify metastases by showing their increased chemical activity compared to that of normal tissues.

An oncologist, radiation oncologist, and surgeon will usually determine the treatment of esophageal cancer, and the oncologist often becomes the primary physician. Treatment sometimes involves neoadjuvant chemotherapy (see chapter 7, "Overview of Colon Cancer"), often combined with radiation therapy.

A gastroenterologist may be involved in several aspects of the care of the patient with esophageal cancer:

- A feeding tube allows for the entrance of formula and medications directly into the stomach, bypassing the tumor in the esophagus, since nutrition can be compromised by a large mass in the esophagus or by the effects of chemotherapy and radiation. These tubes can be placed during an EGD and are easily removed when no longer needed.
- Stage 0 and some stage I tumors can be removed by endoscopic mucosal resection (see earlier section on Barrett's esophagus), often combined with radiofrequency ablation.
- Placement of an expanding metal stent during an EGD is often helpful in keeping the lumen of the esophagus open in patients with more advanced cancers who cannot be treated with surgery or do not respond to chemotherapy and radiation therapy.

The prognosis of esophageal carcinoma has improved in recent years but still remains poor, with a five-year survival of about 15 percent. Many esophageal cancers are advanced by the time they are diagnosed. Prompt attention to trouble swallowing might allow earlier diagnosis and better outcomes in some cases.

TAKE-HOME MESSAGES

- Frequent or daily heartburn should be treated, because there may be serious consequences.
- Sudden, severe chest pain, especially accompanied by dizziness, sweating, shortness of breath, nausea, or palpitations, warrants an immediate trip to the emergency room.
- Heartburn accompanied by trouble swallowing, weight loss, vomiting, black or maroon stools, or anemia should be evaluated promptly.
- Take PPI medications on an empty stomach, thirty to sixty minutes before eating. Make sure you get adequate calcium in your diet. Have your vitamin D, kidney function, and magnesium levels checked periodically.
- PPI medications should not be continued indefinitely in most patients. Ask your doctor when you should stop them or if there is an alternative.
- Surgery for GERD can be an option for some patients with GERD who do not wish to take medications long term or do not respond to medical treatment.

- Barrett's esophagus may progress to esophageal cancer, although most with this disorder will not. A fifty-year-old obese white male with long-standing heartburn who smokes is at very high risk. If some parts of the preceding description fit, prompt evaluation (including EGD) is almost certainly appropriate.
- The outlook of esophageal cancer is improving, especially **when detected early**. Late-stage cancer has a poor prognosis.

15

Disorders of the Stomach and Small Intestine, Including Celiac Disease

This chapter will review five common and important disorders of the stomach: gastroparesis, ulcers, polyps of the stomach, *Helicobacter pylori* infection, and celiac disease. The gluten-free diet for celiac disease is discussed here and also in chapter 19, "Healthy Eating."

GASTROPARESIS

Gastroparesis is a disorder in which the emptying of the stomach is delayed. It is a type of motility disorder, i.e., a disorder of the normal, spontaneous movements of the GI tract. Normally, 50 percent of ingested water will leave the stomach in eight to eighteen minutes; liquids with higher amounts of calories leave the stomach more slowly, and 50 percent of solid food leaves the stomach in two hours. Many solid fats are converted to a liquid by warming to body temperature but nevertheless are emptied more slowly.[1] In gastroparesis, food remains in the stomach longer than normal. Nausea and vomiting are the main symptoms, and they can be long-lasting and severe. In severe cases, less than 10 percent of ingested food may leave the stomach in two hours. Gastroparesis often comes to attention when undigested food is found in the stomach during an upper endoscopy (EGD) despite the patient having followed the instructions regarding not eating after midnight. It is particularly common in people with longstanding diabetes as well as numerous other conditions involving nerve damage, but many people with gastroparesis have no predisposing condition.

The diagnosis is confirmed by a gastric emptying scan, a nuclear medicine test in which the patient eats an egg sandwich containing a stable isotope, following which the stomach is scanned to see how quickly it empties. Gastroparesis is identified by delayed gastric emptying on this test. EGD is usually done to exclude other causes.

Treatment can be challenging. Dietary treatment consists of small meals (up to six per day), more liquids, and reduced fiber. Taking in too much fiber in gastroparesis can lead to a bezoar, a concretion of foreign material which requires removal via EGD or surgery. Some patients benefit from low-fat meals, while others tolerate fat especially in liquid form, which helps provide sufficient calories. Consultation with a dietitian can be helpful. Better control of diabetes, if present, is important. Medications such as metoclopramide and erythromycin can help the stomach empty but can have significant adverse effects. Metaclopramide can cause tremors or other types of abnormal body movements and should be discontinued if these occur. Metoclopramide and erythromycin have potentially serious drug interactions (one drug interfering with the action of another or adding to the toxicity of another) which often limit their use. You should ask about drug interactions if these drugs are prescribed. Amitriptyline, an antidepressant, is sometimes used to modulate symptoms. The pylorus (the lower opening of the stomach) can be injected with Botox, a nerve toxin, in order to promote emptying, but the benefit often disappears after a few weeks or months. Better treatments for this disorder are needed.

GASTRIC AND DUODENAL ULCERS

Ulcers are disruptions in the lining of any part of the GI tract, but this discussion will focus on those in the stomach (figure 15.1) or duodenum. Although once thought to be caused by psychological stress, most gastric (stomach) or duodenal ulcers today are known to be caused by aspirin, non-steroidal anti-inflammatory drugs (NSAIDs: ibuprofen, naproxen, and many others), or a bacteria called *Helicobacter pylori*. Some ulcers have no apparent cause. Ulcers are usually associated with abdominal pain, but many patients with ulcers have no symptoms.

Gastric or duodenal ulcers are most commonly diagnosed at an EGD. They are treated with acid blockers and avoiding NSAIDs; antibiotics are added if *H. pylori* is present (see later in this chapter for more information on *H. pylori*). Bleeding ulcers can usually be treated during an EGD. The initial approach to a bleeding ulcer is to inject epinephrine, a medication that constricts blood vessels, using a catheter with a needle that has been passed through the scope. This usually stops the bleeding temporarily and allows the physician to determine the exact location of the bleeding. Then the bleeding site is either cauterized with a heat probe or closed up with a clip, or both. Surgery is considered if the bleeding cannot be controlled with these methods.

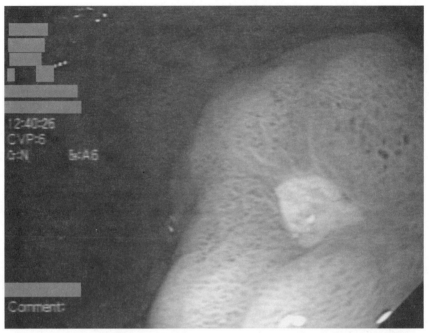

Figure 15.1.   Ulcer in the antrum of the stomach. There is a crater consisting of a clean, white base. This ulcer was associated with NSAID use and did not bleed.
Source: David M. Novick, *Gastric Ulcer*, July 2016.

GASTRIC POLYPS

Gastric polyps are common and almost always benign. It is standard practice to biopsy gastric polyps when they are found in the course of an EGD. Larger polyps, even if hyperplastic, may have a small risk of progressing to cancer. Rarely, an adenoma may be identified in the stomach, and these (like adenomas in the colon) are potentially pre-cancerous. All adenomas and larger hyperplastic polyps should be removed.

Multiple benign gastric polyps, known as fundic gland polyps, are often seen in patients taking PPIs. These have almost no malignant potential.

HELICOBACTER PYLORI (H. PYLORI) INFECTION

H. pylori is a bacteria that can cause peptic ulcer; gastric adenocarcinoma; and a specific type of lymphoma of the stomach, known as MALT lymphoma or low-grade gastric B-cell lymphoma. *H. pylori* resides in the stomach and, in contrast to most bacteria, prefers an acid environment. This bacterium is found in every country of the world and in all age groups, and it is thought to be acquired mainly in childhood. The rate of *H. pylori* infection correlates with socioeconomic status, overcrowding, and poor sanitation. In the United States, the overall incidence of *H. pylori* is decreasing. The incidence of *H. pylori* is increased in gastroenterologists and nurses, probably as a result of exposure to infected fluid or tissue.

H. pylori is the most common cause of duodenal ulcers and is responsible for more than half of the cases in the United States. In non-Western countries, it may cause more than 90 percent of cases. Most patients with *H. pylori* infection do not develop ulcers or any clinically significant digestive problem. *H. pylori* infection may provide a degree of protection against acid reflux (GERD), Barrett's esophagus, and esophageal adenocarcinoma, because the inflammation induced by this bacteria directly reduces gastric output and also damages acid-producing cells of the stomach, further reducing acid production.[2] This reduction in stomach acidity does reduce reflux and its complications, but the effect is not sufficiently strong or consistent to influence treatment decisions.

H. pylori is most commonly diagnosed by a gastric biopsy performed during an EGD. Antibodies to *H. pylori* can be detected by a blood test, but false-positive results occasionally occur.

WHO SHOULD BE TREATED FOR *H. PYLORI*?*

Definite	Probable	Optional
• Gastric ulcer • Duodenal ulcer • MALT lymphoma (low-grade B-cell lymphoma) • Family history of gastric adenocarcinoma	• Long-term NSAID use • Gastric symptoms without ulcers	• No symptoms

*Since most persons infected with *H. pylori* have no clinical consequences, many will not need treatment.

If *H. pylori* is treated with antibiotics, then a test is needed to determine if the bacterium has been eradicated. A stool antigen test or a special breath test is commonly used for this purpose. Follow-up testing should be performed at least one month after the end of treatment, with no PPI medications or antibiotics for any reason for at least two weeks. The *H. pylori* blood test is not useful for follow-up testing because the *H. pylori* antibody persists after treatment. If a follow-up EGD will be done for other reasons, e.g., follow-up of a gastric ulcer to document healing, then a repeat biopsy can document resolution of *H. pylori*.

Treatment of *H. pylori* includes taking at least two antibiotics that have activity against *H. pylori*, along with a twice daily PPI. A relatively small number of antibiotics are effective against *H. pylori*, but bismuth subsalicylate (Pepto-Bismol or others) is also effective. Over the last twenty years, some strains of *H. pylori* have become resistant to the usual antibiotics, and the overall eradication rate has decreased to about 80 percent. Clarithromycin is the most likely antibiotic to be resistant; if you have had recent or multiple treatments with clarithromycin or related antibiotics (erythromycin or azithromycin), an alternative regimen should be used. Most regimens of antibiotics for *H. pylori* require fourteen days of treatment. Strict adherence to the prescribed regimen is advised.

Side effects may occur with all of the medications used for *H. pylori*. If your treatment includes bismuth subsalicylate, do not be surprised if your tongue and your stools turn black; these changes will resolve when the bismuth is stopped. Alcohol must be strictly avoided if your regimen includes metronidazole, as combining these two substances will make you very sick.

CELIAC DISEASE

Celiac disease is characterized by intolerance to gluten, a protein found in wheat, barley, and rye. Celiac disease is common, occurring in about one of 133 people in the United States. It can be diagnosed at any age, including childhood. Celiac disease is an autoimmune disease in which the immune system reacts to gluten, and this reaction leads to damage to the small intestinal wall. Celiac disease can run in families, but the underlying cause is unknown. Some people are sensitive to gluten without having celiac disease, a situation known as gluten sensitivity. This is discussed in chapter 19, "Healthy Eating." Celiac disease is also called celiac sprue or gluten-sensitive enteropathy.

The most common symptoms in adults are diarrhea and weight loss. Abdominal pain and gas are typical complaints. In children, celiac disease may come to attention because of failure to grow or thrive. Some children or adults may have no symptoms or vague complaints that resemble irritable bowel syndrome. Celiac disease can lead to vitamin and mineral deficiencies, including iron, B vitamins, and fat-soluble vitamins (vitamins A, D, E, and K). Iron deficiency anemia and osteopenia (thinning of bones) can result. People with unexplained iron deficiency anemia should be evaluated for celiac disease.

Celiac disease is associated with certain other medical conditions:

MEDICAL DISORDERS ASSOCIATED WITH CELIAC DISEASE

- Type 1 diabetes mellitus
- Thyroid problems
- Abnormal liver test results
- Down syndrome
- Dermatitis herpetiformis—A rash with blisters that is rare but strongly associated with celiac disease

---

Celiac disease, especially if untreated, can lead to cancer of the small intestine. This is one of the reasons why strict adherence to a gluten-free diet (see section later in this chapter) is essential for people with this condition.

The diagnosis of celiac disease is made by a biopsy of the small intestine, done during an EGD, and by observing improvement of symptoms, blood test results, and biopsy findings with a gluten-free diet. The small intestinal biopsy of a celiac patient shows increased numbers of lymphocytes (a common type of white blood cell) in the lining of the intestine, and blunting or flattening of the villi (the normal projections of the surface of the intestine). The initial test performed is usually a blood test for relevant antibodies, the most important of which is tissue transglutaminase, and is positive in about 90 percent of celiac patients. EGD or wireless capsule endoscopy may reveal scalloped folds or a cracked-earth pattern. If celiac disease is diagnosed, then testing of first-degree relatives (parents, siblings, and children) is advisable.

The antibody tests and small intestinal biopsies are best done on a **regular** diet, not gluten-free. A gluten-free diet can normalize the blood and biopsy results. Therefore, if you think that you might have celiac disease, get tested before starting a gluten-free diet.

When a patient who is already on a gluten-free diet requests celiac testing, or when the antibody test results are indefinite, a blood test for certain genetic markers (HLA-DQ2 and HLA-DQ8) may be helpful. This test can rule out celiac disease with 97 percent accuracy but cannot rule it in.

Celiac disease is treated with a lifelong gluten-free diet. The diet is challenging for some patients, especially in the beginning, but strict adherence is essential to prevent symptoms and complications. Consultation with a dietitian may be helpful.

When a patient with celiac disease does not respond to a gluten-free diet, the most likely reason is that he or she is unknowingly ingesting gluten or is cheating. It is necessary to exclude **all** gluten from the diet. Other possible reasons for persistent symptoms while adhering to a gluten-free diet include the following:

- Refractory celiac disease, i.e., celiac disease that does not respond to a gluten-free diet and in which no other explanation can be found.[3] This may respond to corticosteroid treatment.[4]
- Other food intolerances
  - FODMAPS: See glossary for definition and chapter 9, "Irritable Bowel Syndrome," for details.
  - Fructose
  - Lactose
  - Soy
  - Oats (see discussion later in this chapter)
- Coexisting irritable bowel syndrome or microscopic colitis
- Cancer of the small intestine, usually a lymphoma

THE GLUTEN-FREE DIET

Gluten is found in wheat, barley, and rye. Oats in pure form do not contain gluten, but they are frequently contaminated with wheat in the food-manufacturing process. It is best to avoid oats initially when celiac disease is diagnosed. Gluten-free oats can be gradually introduced when the patient with celiac disease is stable and responding to the gluten-free diet. Most celiac patients can tolerate gluten-free oats.

Although a gluten-free diet may seem restrictive at first, there are a large number of foods that are allowed, as shown in the box below.

FOODS THAT ARE ALLOWED IN THE GLUTEN-FREE DIET

- Fresh meat, fish, and poultry*
- Seeds and nuts (unprocessed)
- Legumes
- Eggs
- Fruits

- Vegetables
- Potatoes
- Corn
- Rice
- Most dairy products

*Not breaded or marinated.

How do you know if a food is gluten-free? Recently, the U.S. Food and Drug Administration (FDA), which has jurisdiction over packaged foods, ruled that in order for a food to be labeled *gluten-free*, it must contain no wheat, barley, or rye. If it contains an ingredient that is derived from a gluten-containing grain, from which gluten has been removed, then it must contain less than twenty parts per million of gluten.[5] This rule also covers dietary supplements.

The U.S. Department of Agriculture (USDA) regulates meat, poultry, and eggs. The USDA encourages voluntary compliance with the rule set forth by the FDA, as does the Alcohol and Tobacco Tax and Trade Bureau. All of these agencies intend to avoid misleading claims, and have drafted statements endorsing the spirit of the FDA rule. Nevertheless, for consumers, caution is always advisable.

One of the difficulties of maintaining a gluten-free diet is that wheat products come in many forms, with different names. The two boxes below show products that should be avoided by celiac patients unless marked gluten-free.

GRAIN PRODUCTS THAT CONTAIN GLUTEN AND SHOULD BE AVOIDED*

- Couscous
- Durum
- Farina
- Farro
- Graham flour
- Matzah
- Semolina
- Spelt

*Also beware of crossbred hybrid grains such as triticale,[6] a cross between wheat and rye; such products may contain gluten.

UNEXPECTED GLUTEN-CONTAINING PRODUCTS*

- Beer
- Flavored rice
- French fries
- Gravy
- Pasta
- Potato chips
- Processed foods
- Salad dressing
- Soups
- Soy sauce and other sauces
- Tortilla

*Unless labeled gluten-free.

Fortunately, there are a number of grains or grain substitutes that do not contain gluten.[7] Many of these can be substituted for grains in recipes:

GRAINS OR GRAIN SUBSTITUTES THAT DO NOT CONTAIN GLUTEN

- Amaranth
- Arrowroot
- Buckwheat
- Corn
- Cassava
- Flax
- Millet
- Quinoa
- Rice
- Sorghum
- Soy
- Tapioca
- Teff

It is important to note that processed foods made from the above grains are not necessarily enriched with iron, folic acid, or other B vitamins; that is, they may be made from refined grains.[8] Many dietitians recommend using whole grains or whole-grain flours.

EATING GLUTEN-FREE AWAY FROM HOME[9-11]

Eating gluten-free in restaurants or in other peoples' homes can be a rewarding experience if sufficient planning is done. One of the greatest risks in either situation is **cross contamination**: the inadvertent mixing of gluten-containing and gluten-free food. Cross contamination could occur when the same spatula is used to flip hamburgers and buns, when the food preparer uses the same gloves to prepare gluten-containing and gluten-free food, or when the same serving spoon is used for the gluten-free salad and the salad with croutons. Since some celiac patients react severely to tiny amounts of gluten, it is important to try to avoid eating in places where cross contamination is likely. Another hazard is the lack of knowledge about celiac disease. Some servers or restaurant managers may say that they can prepare gluten-free food but do not take all the necessary precautions. Websites of celiac organizations and smartphone apps (Find Me Gluten Free, Gluten Free Registry, and others) can be very helpful in finding gluten-free restaurants.

The ideal gluten-free dining will be at a restaurant where there is a separate, dedicated area for gluten-free food preparation. There will be dedicated pots and pans, and French fries will be made in a separate fryer.

STEPS FOR FRUITFUL GLUTEN-FREE DINING

- Check the restaurant's website and review the menu.
- Ask for a gluten-free menu.
- Call ahead and speak to the manager.
- See if the restaurant has a certification from a celiac organization.
- Ask a lot of questions and assess the willingness and knowledge to make the meal truly gluten-free.
- Tell your server that you cannot have anything with wheat, barley, rye, or oats.
- Look on the menu for more simple or plain items.
- Avoid fried foods and ask for no croutons on salads.
- Pay close attention to toppings and sauces.
- Ask that the grill be cleaned before your item is cooked.

Fast-food restaurants are particularly challenging because they have a limited menu and may not be able to make changes, but the above steps can be used for fast food as well. One advantage of fast-food restaurants, however, is that from inside the restaurant you can see right into the kitchen, and you can make an assessment. Drive-thru restaurants are riskier. At all restaurants, buffets and salad bars have a high risk of cross contamination and are best avoided.

Dining at someone's home may be easier but is not without pitfalls. It's advisable to assess the willingness of your host or hostess to meet your needs. If he or she is responsive, explain the concept of cross contamination. Bring a disposable serving spoon to the meal and explain why. You can also offer to bring part or all of your own meal or suggest some simple items that are less likely to become contaminated.

CASE REPORT: DID YOU BRING SOME KIND OF BUG INTO THE HOUSE?

Walt, forty-five, and his daughter, Jen, fifteen, both developed small itching blisters on and around both elbows. When Walt realized that they both had the same rash, he said, "What kind of bug did you bring into the house? I told you I don't like you hanging around with your friend Jessica in the woods next to the park!"

"Jessie has nothing to do with this," Jen replied, rolling her eyes. "I haven't seen any bugs, and if there were, Mom would have your rash," she said while walking out of the room.

Jen's mom took her to the pediatrician, who diagnosed psoriasis. Walt saw his family doctor, who also thought it was psoriasis. In both cases, the rash got better initially but kept coming back. It was itchy and burning, and it was hard to stop scratching. Walt sometimes had to change his shirt at work because of bleeding by the elbows.

Finally, Walt went to a dermatologist, who looked at the rash for what seemed like a long time. She said, "I know what this is, but we need to confirm it with a skin biopsy. It is called dermatitis herpetiformis."

"It's herpes?" Walt blurted out.

"No, not at all. It is actually a sign of celiac disease. When you are done with me, you will need to see a gastroenterologist."

Walt and Jen both had positive blood tests and small intestinal biopsies, confirming the diagnosis of celiac disease. Although they struggled with the gluten-free diet at first, the dermatitis herpetiformis resolved, and they are now great fans of quinoa, amaranth, and buckwheat.

TAKE-HOME MESSAGES

- Gastroparesis, a condition in which the stomach does not empty normally, is treated with small meals, control of diabetes, a low-fiber diet, and medications.
- Metoclopramide is helpful for many patients with gastroparesis but must be stopped immediately if tremors or abnormal body movements are observed.
- Celiac disease comes to medical attention because of diarrhea, weight loss, abdominal pain, and/or gas. It should be considered in patients with unexplained iron deficiency anemia.
- Untreated celiac disease can lead to cancer of the small intestine. Lifelong adherence to the gluten-free diet is strongly recommended.
- Cross contamination, the inadvertent mixing of gluten-containing and gluten-free food, is a major barrier to celiac patients' ability to eat in restaurants or other people's homes. With careful planning, gluten-free dining in these settings is possible.

16

Gallbladder and Pancreas

Bile, a mixture of substances that aid in digestion, is made in the liver and travels down a network of bile ducts to reach the gallbladder, where it is stored until needed. After someone eats, the gallbladder contracts in response to food reaching certain parts of the GI tract and releases bile into the small intestine. Bile reaches the small intestine via the common bile duct, which has a common opening with the pancreatic duct; this opening is known as the ampulla of Vater (see diagram 3 before chapter 1). The muscle at the ampulla of Vater is called the sphincter of Oddi, and it controls when bile or pancreatic juices enter the small intestine. The structure consisting of the openings of pancreatic and bile ducts and the regulatory sphincter is called the major papilla. The pancreas has a small amount of drainage from a minor papilla as well.

GALLSTONES (CHOLELITHIASIS)

Gallstones consist primarily of either cholesterol or bilirubin, a substance produced during the breakdown of heme, a component of red blood cells. Gallstones found in people without symptoms who are undergoing CT scan, ultrasound, or other tests for an unrelated reason are referred to as "incidental gallstones." They require no treatment.

About three-fourths of people with gallstones have no problem, but the stones in the remainder can have the following effects:

- Block the outflow from the gallbladder, potentially causing inflammation of the gallbladder (cholecystitis)

- Block the bile ducts, potentially causing jaundice and sometimes infections in the bile ducts (cholangitis)
- Block the pancreatic ducts, potentially causing inflammation of the pancreas (pancreatitis)

RISK FACTORS FOR GALLSTONES

- Female
- Older age
- Obesity
- Estrogen treatment
- Very rapid weight loss

- Diabetes mellitus
- Pregnancy
- Ethnicity*
- Sickle cell anemia**

*Increased in whites, Hispanics, and especially Native Americans. Decreased in African Americans.
**Associated with bilirubin stones. Most others have cholesterol stones.

The following sections will detail some of the common syndromes associated with gallbladder disease. It should be kept in mind that there are many atypical presentations of gallbladder disease, which always warrant consideration when the diagnosis is not clear.

BILIARY COLIC

The typical gallbladder pain is known as biliary colic, which is a misnomer because it's more often a dull, steady pain (colic increases and decreases in intensity during an attack). Biliary colic can result when the gallbladder contracts while there is a stone blocking the exit. Located in the right middle or upper abdomen, biliary colic may extend to the right shoulder or back. It's usually associated with nausea and vomiting. The intensity can be anywhere from mild to severe. It is not worse with movement. Biliary colic lasts for one to four hours and often follows a meal, especially a fatty one.

Evaluation includes laboratory tests; ultrasound; and, most importantly, exclusion of other causes. An EGD is often done to exclude ulcer disease and other upper GI disease states. Treatment is the surgical removal of the gallbladder (cholecystectomy) after a careful assessment of the benefits and risks. A patient with mild symptoms but high surgical risk due to other medical conditions may be best managed by close observation. Cholecystectomy is done using a laparoscope when possible, which involves three or four small incisions in the abdomen through which cameras and tools are inserted. This technique is associated with reduced post-operative pain and a shorter hospital stay in comparison to the "open" procedure in which a much longer incision is made and the surgeon uses his hands, scalpels, and scissors to remove the gallbladder.

ACUTE CHOLECYSTITIS

Acute cholecystitis is manifested by right upper and mid upper abdominal pain that is more prolonged and severe than that of biliary colic. The pain may radiate to the right shoulder or back.

If you have "gallbladder pain" lasting more than four hours and it's not getting better, go to the hospital emergency room. Early diagnosis leads to better outcomes.

The pain is associated with fever, nausea, and vomiting, and in contrast to biliary colic, it is worse with movement. On examination, the patient appears ill and often has a rapid heart rate and elevation in the white blood cell count. Ultrasound typically shows gallstones, thickening of the gallbladder wall, and fluid around the gallbladder.

MURPHY'S SIGN*

While examining the patient, the doctor observes the patient's breathing and then places his or her hands on the right upper abdomen near the lower ribs. Murphy's sign is present when in response to this pressure the patient abruptly stops breathing in. Murphy's sign can also be elicited by an ultrasound probe being placed on the right upper abdomen and observing the cessation of inspiration. This is called the *sonographic Murphy's sign*.

*Not to be confused with Murphy's Law, which is "anything that can go wrong will go wrong." Murphy's Law comes into play in medicine, as evidenced by the complications discussed later in this chapter, but it can be foiled by prompt diagnosis and treatment.

There are, of course, many other causes of abdominal pain, the sorting out of which requires considerable skill. The next step, if the diagnosis is in doubt, is often a nuclear medicine scan of the gallbladder, commonly known as a HIDA scan. During a HIDA scan, a chemical is injected through an intravenous (IV) catheter. This chemical can be detected by a special nuclear imaging camera, usually located in the radiology department. Normally the chemical is processed by the liver, excreted in the bile, and filled into the gallbladder. A second chemical, called cholecystokinin (CCK), is often administered to stimulate the gallbladder to contract and excrete the bile into the intestine. In acute cholecystitis, the gallbladder does not visualize on a HIDA scan because the outflow of the gallbladder is blocked by stones or inflammation. The blockage can be at the exit of the gallbladder or the cystic duct, which connects the gallbladder to the common bile duct and through which bile exits the gallbladder (see diagram 3 before chapter 1). Other testing may be done depending on the clinical circumstances. Making the diagnosis is important because there are several serious complications of acute cholecystitis that include the following:

- Emphysematous cholecystitis: inflammation of the gallbladder with gas-forming bacteria.
- Gangrene of the gallbladder: infection complicated by insufficient blood supply, extensive tissue death, and putrefaction (decomposition of tissue which becomes liquid and has a noxious odor).
- Gallstone pancreatitis: inflammation of the pancreas caused by a stone at the ampulla of Vater (see section on "Acute Pancreatitis").
- Gallstone ileus: the situation when a gallstone has passed out of the gallbladder, through the cystic duct, common bile duct, and ampulla of Vater, and into the small intestine. The stone causes an intestinal obstruction, usually at the junction between the small and large intestine.

Treatment of the hospitalized patient with acute cholecystitis includes IV fluids, antibiotics, pain control, surgical consultation, and cholecystectomy. The timing of the cholecystectomy depends greatly on the severity of the acute disease and any coexisting medical problems that increase the risk of surgery. Treatment of the non-hospitalized patient with acute cholecystitis involves convincing the patient to go to the hospital.

COMMON BILE DUCT STONE (CHOLEDOCHOLITHIASIS)

Gallstones that exit the gallbladder and traverse the cystic duct will enter the common bile duct, which leads directly to the small intestine. Gallstones can lodge in the common bile duct or at the ampulla of Vater, where the common bile duct enters the small intestine, along with the pancreatic duct. They can also form directly in the common bile duct, even after the gallbladder has been removed. Common duct stones can be found in patients with biliary colic or acute cholecystitis. Most commonly, they present with right upper abdominal pain, nausea, or vomiting, but in some patients there are no symptoms. Common duct stones may come to attention because of abnormal liver blood tests; dilated biliary ducts on ultrasound or CT scan; or jaundice, a yellow discoloration of the white parts of the eyes or of the skin. In the latter situation, jaundice occurs because of the backup of bile behind the obstructing stone. Common duct stones can cause pancreatitis or cholangitis (bile duct infection, with fever and elevated white cell count).

Several additional tests or procedures can be done for diagnosis and treatment of common duct stones, as well as for other disorders of the liver, gallbladder, bile ducts, and pancreas:

- MRCP, or magnetic resonance cholangiopancreatography: A form of magnetic resonance imaging (MRI) that can image the biliary and pancreatic ducts. MRCP is usually the next test done for common duct stones after ultrasound or CT.
- EUS, or endoscopic ultrasound: The ultrasound probe on the tip of the scope can get very close to the relevant structures and can provide detailed imaging. If a mass is found, a type of biopsy called fine-needle aspiration, or FNA, can be done. In FNA, a very thin needle is used to withdraw cells. The needle is so thin that it can go through the wall of the small intestine without causing injury.
- ERCP, or endoscopic retrograde cholangiopancreatography: While this procedure can provide important images of the biliary or pancreatic ducts, its main importance is as a therapeutic procedure. It's done with a specialized upper endoscope, known as a duodenoscope, with side-viewing rather than forward-viewing lenses; these lenses directly view the walls of the GI tract rather than the lumen, and provide an excellent view of the papilla, which contains the ampulla of Vater and the sphincter of Oddi. During the ERCP, a tube can be placed into the common bile duct or pancreatic duct to inject contrast for imaging, stones can be removed by various devices that are passed through the scope, an incision can be made in the sphincter of Oddi (sphincterotomy) to allow easier exit of stones, and a stent can be placed to prevent reobstruction if further stones remain that cannot be removed at that time. ERCP is an invasive test that has risks, most commonly pancreatitis (5–20 percent of patients), and rarely perforation or bleeding. See chapter 13, "Evaluation of the Esophagus, Stomach, and Small Intestine," for discussion of episodes of infection transmitted during ERCP. Post-ERCP pancreatitis can be mild to severe, but there are techniques to reduce the risk. Very rarely, complications from ERCP can lead to death.

- Intraoperative cholangiogram: Injection of contrast during cholecystectomy to image the biliary system.

Treatment of common duct stones is removal by ERCP. Surgical removal is rarely needed and carries more risk than ERCP. For those patients whose gallbladder is still present, cholecystectomy is often recommended, especially when there are stones remaining within the gallbladder.

FUNCTIONAL GALLBLADDER DISEASE

This entity is characterized by biliary-type pain with no gallstones. Other causes of abdominal pain must be excluded.

FEATURES OF PAIN THAT SUGGEST FUNCTIONAL GALLBLADDER DISEASE[1,2]

- Right or mid upper abdominal pain, with or without nausea
- Recurrent episodes (but not every day), most commonly after a fatty meal
- Pain for thirty minutes or longer
- Pain that interferes with daily life
- Pain that is not relieved by antacids, changes in position, or having a bowel movement

---

If all of the above are present, a nuclear medicine gallbladder scan (HIDA scan) is appropriate. During scanning, the hormone CCK is injected and causes the gallbladder to contract. The percentage of the gallbladder contents that is expelled by this contraction, known as the gallbladder ejection fraction, is calculated. Patients with ejection fractions less than 35 percent are likely to respond well to cholecystectomy.

THE PANCREAS

The pancreas provides enzymes that digest food and bicarbonate to neutralize acid entering the first part of the duodenum from the stomach. It is also important in fat digestion. It is stimulated by food and by hormones originating in the GI tract. Pancreatic enzymes are released into the small intestine via a duct system, with the main pancreatic duct joining the common bile duct at the ampulla of Vater. The cells producing digestive enzymes and bicarbonate are known as *exocrine* cells; that is, they secrete internally via a duct. The pancreas also has *endocrine* (hormone-producing) cells that produce insulin for control of blood glucose, as well as several other hormones.

ACUTE PANCREATITIS

Acute pancreatitis is an inflamed pancreas characterized by intense abdominal pain. Acute pancreatitis is among the most common gastrointestinal reasons for admission to the hospital. While about 80 percent of patients recover in three to five days with an uneventful course, the remainder can have prolonged hospital stays with complications, some of which can lead to necrosis, or cell death. In severe cases, the death rate for acute pancreatitis is 10–30 percent, depending on the type of patients selected for analysis.

CAUSES OF ACUTE PANCREATITIS

Top Two	Others	Major Risk Factor
• Gallstones	• Elevated triglycerides	• Smoking
• Alcohol	• Trauma	
	• Medications*	
	• Post-ERCP	
	• Any cause of elevated blood calcium	
	• Pancreatic or ampulla of Vater tumor	
	• Heredity	
	• Scorpion bites	
	• Unknown	

*Including diuretics, sulfa drugs, azathioprine, 6-mercaptopurine, and corticosteroids.

The abdominal pain is sudden and severe. It frequently extends to the back, and it is somewhat alleviated by sitting up and leaning forward. The pain is associated with nausea, vomiting, and shortness of breath. It is intense enough to bring the patient to the hospital.

On examination, the patient appears ill. Rapid heart rate, low blood pressure, low oxygen saturation, and fever can be present. Jaundice may be present, usually a result of bile duct obstruction from a gallstone. The mid to upper abdomen is tender. An elevation of the pancreatic enzymes and amylase and lipase on blood testing leads to the diagnosis, and it is confirmed by CT scan of the abdomen, done optimally with contrast. In cases where the diagnosis is clear because of physical exam and blood tests, a CT scan may not be necessary. Ultrasound is less useful because the pancreas can be obscured by bowel gas. EUS can be helpful when the cause is not clear.

In the patient who does not recover quickly, a number of complications can be seen:

- Fluid collections.
- Pseudocyst: a fluid collection surrounded by inflammation. It's not a true cyst as it has no wall. While most pseudocysts have no symptoms, some can cause pain, impinge on the small intestine or bile ducts, or become infected.
- Necrotizing pancreatitis: pancreatitis with inflammation and necrosis, or cell death. When necrotizing pancreatitis is present, a CT scan shows that the pancreas does not take up the contrast. This may not be seen on the initial CT scan but may be well documented on a CT scan with contrast done three to seven days after the onset of symptoms.[3]
- Worsening of preexisting conditions such as heart or lung disease.
- Systemic inflammatory response syndrome (SIRS): persistent abnormalities in heart rate, respiratory rate, body temperature, and white blood cell count. The presence of SIRS on admission or forty-eight hours after admission predicts severe disease.[4]
- Organ failure.

Treatment of the hospitalized patient with acute pancreatitis is complex and depends greatly on the individual circumstances. The initial treatment is large-volume intravenous fluid (nothing by mouth) and pain control. For mild cases, feedings are started when the pain abates. Initial feedings are clear liquids, gradually advanced to a soft, low-fat diet. Nutritional support is often recommended if the hospital stay goes beyond five days, and the preferred method is a temporary feeding tube that enters the nose and extends to the small intestine. Antibiotics are used if infection is documented or strongly suspected. ERCP is indicated to treat bile duct obstruction from gallstones. Sicker patients are treated in an intensive care unit, and the hospital stay can be of long duration. Cholecystectomy is recommended after recovery from gallstone pancreatitis, including patients with crystals or tiny stones in the bile, i.e., gallbladder sludge.

CHRONIC PANCREATITIS

Longstanding (chronic) inflammation of the pancreas can lead to digestive difficulties or chronic pain. These changes, which can be permanent and are associated with deposits of scar tissue in the pancreas, are known as chronic pancreatitis.

The pain in chronic pancreatitis is typically in the mid upper abdomen. It may be intermittent or continuous, and may radiate to the back. The pain can be severe and can lead to dependence on prescription opioids. Some patients have no pain.

Chronic pancreatitis is also associated with problems with digestion because the pancreas can no longer make sufficient amounts of digestive enzymes. The inability to digest fat leads to loose, greasy, or oily stools. Deficiencies in fat-soluble vitamins (vitamins A, D, E, and K) may occur. With loss of the endocrine cells of the pancreas, insulin-dependent diabetes mellitus may also develop.

Complications include pseudocysts, pancreatic duct leaks that connect to the abdominal cavity or the lung lining and lead to fluid buildup in these areas (known as pancreatic ascites and pancreatic pleural effusion, respectively), and pancreatic cancer. X-rays sometimes show calcium deposits in the pancreas.

Excessive alcohol use is the most common cause of chronic pancreatitis in men and one of the causes in women. Chronic pancreatitis is of unknown cause in most patients without alcoholism. Smoking is also a contributing factor. There is conflicting evidence that nutritional deficiencies, especially of antioxidants, may play a role.

Initial treatment is discontinuing alcohol use and treatment of bile duct obstruction, if these are present. Pain management can be challenging and may require involvement of a pain management specialist. Small, low-fat meals are recommended. Medium-chain triglycerides may be absorbed better than other fats, and supplements are available. Supplements of fat-soluble vitamins can be used. Pancreatic enzymes can be taken in a pill form to assist with digestion. There are surgical procedures for chronic pancreatitis that have helped some patients and should be considered when medical management fails. A careful evaluation of the risks and benefits is essential. Consultation with a surgeon experienced in these procedures is recommended.

PANCREATIC CANCER

Adenocarcinoma of the pancreas (the main type of pancreatic cancer) is among the most dire diagnoses that a gastroenterologist can make. It is almost always incurable and is the fourth leading cause of cancer death in the United States. Surgical cure rates are less than 5 percent, and chemotherapy is minimally effective. People with pancreatic cancer should take a very cautious approach when any doctor claims good results for a treatment, especially a new and unproven one. A way to detect this lethal disease at an early stage, in which the prognosis might be better, is urgently needed.

RISK FACTORS FOR PANCREATIC ADENOCARCINOMA

- Chronic pancreatitis
- Diabetes mellitus

- Smoking
- Obesity

Adenocarcinoma of the pancreas arises from the exocrine cells of the pancreas that produce digestive enzymes and bicarbonate. Weight loss, fatigue, and loss of appetite are common initial symptoms. Abdominal pain is common, though some patients present with painless jaundice. Jaundice is most common when the tumor is near the bile ducts (the head of the pancreas) and may not be present when the tumor is farther away. Nausea, back pain, and diarrhea are additional symptoms.

Physical examination may reveal jaundice or a mass in the abdomen. The diagnosis is challenging and complex, and it varies tremendously based on individual circumstances. Ultrasound or CT are usually the initial tests. EUS is often done next if the diagnosis of pancreatic cancer is suspected but not found, as EUS can detect smaller tumors that may be missed by ultrasound or CT; such small tumors may be less likely to have metastasized. FNA during EUS can confirm the diagnosis if a tumor is seen. MRCP may be done if ERCP is not technically possible, e.g., when the scope cannot reach the ampulla of Vater because of previous gastric surgery or when there is an obstruction at the outflow to the stomach. ERCP is done more often for a therapeutic intervention than for diagnosis. It is very useful for placing stents or guide wires for stents when the tumor causes bile duct obstruction. For diagnostic purposes, EUS is more accurate for obtaining samples and has fewer complications than ERCP.

One test that is not useful in the initial evaluation is the CA 19-9, which, like the carcinoembryonic antigen (CEA) (see chapter 7, "Overview of Colon Cancer"), is erroneously referred to as a tumor marker. CA 19-9 is not a useful diagnostic test but has some value in gauging response to treatment if the initial level is high. Similarly, there is no evidence that any sort of screening test for pancreatic cancer is useful for the average patient. Screening with EUS or MRCP may have some role in very high-risk individuals who have, e.g., multiple blood relatives with pancreatic cancer or known genetic predisposition for pancreatic cancer, but more research is needed.[5]

The most important aspect of staging of pancreatic adenocarcinoma is to identify the small number of patients that have a chance for a surgical cure; that is, the cancer is localized, can be completely removed, and has not metastasized. The tumor will be considered unresectable (i.e., surgical cure is not possible) if it has spread to lymph nodes or other organs, or if it has invaded any of the several large blood vessels in the area. Underlying this assessment is the desire to spare the patient an unnecessary major operation. All of the imaging procedures described previously can be helpful in this determination. In some borderline cases, a laparoscopy (during which the abdominal organs can be viewed directly using a scope that is placed through a small incision) can be helpful.

For the small number of patients in whom surgery for pancreatic adenocarcinoma with intent to cure is undertaken, the type of procedure depends on the location of the tumor within the pancreas. Cancers of the head of the pancreas are treated with one of several forms of the Whipple procedure, which involves removal of the affected part of the pancreas, the upper or proximal small intestine (including the duodenum and beginning of the jejunum), common bile duct, gallbladder, and part of the stomach. Tumors of the distal pancreas (pancreatic body or tail) are less commonly resectable than those of the pancreatic head, because they do not block the common bile duct leading to jaundice; they are associated with fewer symptoms and are diagnosed at more advanced stages. When surgery is attempted, the affected part of the pancreas is removed along with the spleen. Most patients with adenocarcinoma of the pancreas are not cured with surgery because microscopic metastases have already taken place.

CASE REPORT: SOMETIMES YOU ONLY GET ONE CHANCE.

Mr. Bourey Son, a sixty-year-old Cambodian man, came in for mild midabdominal pain. He had slight nausea but no weight loss, GI bleeding, fever, or jaundice. He was not taking any medication and had no other medical problems. Physical examination was normal. A CT scan revealed a 1.5-centimeter (about 5/8-inch) mass in the body of the pancreas. MRCP was normal. EUS confirmed the mass and showed no abnormal lymph nodes. FNA of the mass was positive for adenocarcinoma.

Dr. Marks saw Mr. Son in the office and reviewed the findings. The patient spoke little English, and his daughter, Dara, translated. The patient's wife had died of hepatocellular carcinoma a few years ago. Dr. Marks was thinking about how rare a surgical cure of pancreatic carcinoma was and that he had never personally seen such a case.

"There is a definite chance that you can be cured with surgery, because the cancer is small and there is no evidence that it has spread. But to have the best odds of a cure, I advise you to have the surgery as soon as possible. We don't know exactly how much time we have, but these tumors are usually incurable. This may be the rare exception."

Dr. Marks watched Mr. Son as his daughter translated, but Mr. Son's expression revealed little.

Dara said, "My father thanks you for everything that you have done. But he wants to go back to our home country, to see his family. Also, there are some traditional medicines that he wants to try."

Dr. Marks tried a few counterarguments, but to no avail. Mr. Son left for Cambodia within the week.

One year later, Mr. Son returned to Dr. Marks's office. His eyes and skin had turned yellow. His appetite was poor, and he had lost fifteen pounds. Physical examination showed jaundice and a mass in the upper mid-abdomen. CT scan, MRCP, and EUS indicated that the mass had spread to lymph nodes and had eroded into a large blood vessel, and the cancer was deemed unresectable. He passed away four months later.

TAKE-HOME MESSAGES

- Gallstones are common and cause no problems in most people.
- Typical gallbladder pain (biliary colic) is a dull, steady pain in the right or mid upper abdomen, frequently associated with nausea and vomiting.
- There are many atypical presentations of gallstones or gallbladder disease.
- Gallbladder pain lasting more than four hours, especially if it's getting worse, warrants a visit to the hospital emergency room.
- Stones in the common bile duct can often be removed by ERCP.
- ERCP is very useful for removing stones or bypassing obstructions of the bile ducts, but ERCP-induced pancreatitis is not rare. There are techniques to reduce the risk.
- Acute pancreatitis can be mild or severe, and the latter has a high complication and mortality rate.
- Adenocarcinoma of the pancreas is rarely cured by surgery and never by chemotherapy or other treatments. A way to diagnose this disorder at an early stage is urgently needed.

17

Hepatitis C

In the 1960s, vast cultural changes took place in the United States and to varying degrees around the world: a new interest in exploring the limits of consciousness and perception, and a new emphasis on righting injustices. There was a rejection of the conformity that characterized the 1950s and a reexamination of commonly held assumptions. An example of the latter was the idea that marijuana was a "gateway drug" that would reliably lead to addiction to heroin or other dangerous drugs. Once enough people had tried marijuana for various reasons and concluded that the link between marijuana and heroin was not there, at least some began to question the stringencies attached to other drugs, including intravenous heroin. A tremendous increase in experimentation with heroin (and many other drugs) ensued in the latter 1960s and 1970s. Many of these new heroin users decided that it wasn't for them and moved on, while some became addicted. As a result of use of contaminated needles, most people who tried heroin by injection were infected with the hepatitis C virus (HCV), an organism that was unknown at the time. Other people were infected by blood transfusions, which were not screened as well as they are today.

Subsequent surveys of the health of Americans revealed a tremendous increase in the prevalence of HCV in people born between 1945 and 1965 (the baby boomer generation) compared with those born before or after.[1] Based on these observations, it is recommended that **anyone born between 1945 and 1965 should be tested for hepatitis C**.[2] This test is covered by Medicare.

It was estimated based on these health surveys that 2.7 million people in the United States have chronic (long-lasting) HCV infection.[3] The true

135

number is higher because incarcerated or homeless people, who are more likely to be infected with HCV, were not included. **At least half of those with HCV infection do not know that they have it.** At least 60 percent of people with HCV infection acquired it from injection drug use,[4] and this is also likely an underestimate because people often do not admit to their history of drug use, especially if it was a long time ago. The proportion of HCV patients resulting from drug use will increase because of the heroin epidemic of the 2010s.[5,6] Even a single drug injection can transmit HCV.

Other factors associated with an increased frequency of HCV infection are:

- Incarcerated (ever)
- Nasal use of drugs (snorting)
- Long-term hemodialysis for kidney failure
- Tattoo not done professionally
- Health care or emergency service personnel who have needlestick injuries
- Children born to HCV-positive mother (5 percent risk)
- Blood transfusion before 1992
- Human immunodeficiency virus (HIV) infection
- Elevated liver enzymes

> If you have any risk factor for HCV, even if the events occurred a long time ago, get tested.

HCV is rarely transmitted sexually. In my experience, if the partner of a patient with HCV infection has not used drugs, he or she will test negative for HCV. Studies suggest that the same strain of HCV is found in only 2 percent of heterosexual couples in which one partner had no HCV risk factors.[7] The question of failure to disclose drug use history is relevant to these studies also. One exception is in men who have sex with men when one partner is infected with HIV and HCV; sexual transmission is increased in this setting.[8]

"I HAVE HEPATITIS C. HOW CAN I AVOID SPREADING IT?"

- Do not share a razor, toothbrush, nail scissors, or similar grooming tools that could conceivably lead to bleeding.
- If you are bleeding, attend to it yourself if at all possible, or warn the person trying to help you to wear gloves or wash their hands immediately after helping you.
- Do not inject drugs (except for those prescribed by a doctor along with clean syringes and needles). If you have a drug problem, seek help.
- HCV is not spread by sneezing; coughing; or sharing utensils, drinking glasses, food, or water. It is not spread by mosquitos. Quarantine is not needed.
- "Safe sex" precautions are not needed for monogamous heterosexual couples. You should use precautions such as condoms, dental dams, or gloves with a new partner.
- Men who have sex with men who have HCV and HIV should practice safe sex.

THE HEPATITIS C VIRUS

HCV is one of the five common viruses of which hepatitis (inflammation of the liver) is the main consequence. Hepatitis B is more common worldwide but, because of vaccination over the last twenty-five years, is becoming very uncommon in the United States except in immigrants. Hepatitis D requires the presence of hepatitis B and is also prevented by hepatitis B vaccination. Hepatitis A causes acute but not chronic hepatitis and is vaccine preventable. Hepatitis E causes acute hepatitis in healthy people but can become chronic in immunocompromised persons. Hepatitis E is likely to be vaccine preventable in the near future.

A hallmark of HCV is genetic variability, meaning that HCV is really a group of related viruses.[9] Hepatitis C viruses differ from each other in two major ways: genotypes and quasispecies. There are six major genotypes, or strains, numbered 1–6, that are divided into subtypes. A genotype 7 was added to the classification in 2014.[10] They may differ from each other by up to one third of their nucleotide sequence (nucleotides are the "building blocks" of viruses). There are more than fifty subtypes of HCV. In the United States, genotype 1 is the most common, and most of these are subtypes 1a or 1b. In a recent study, the distribution of genotypes was as follows:[11]

- Genotype 1a: 36.3 percent
- Genotype 1b: 23.7 percent

- Other genotype 1: 10 percent
- Genotype 2: 16.2 percent
- Genotype 3: 11.8 percent
- Genotype 4: 1.14 percent
- Genotype 5: 0.03 percent
- Genotype 6: 0.91 percent

Genotypes and subtypes influence the progression of liver disease and the response to antiviral therapy. For example, genotype 3 causes more rapid progression of liver disease than genotypes 1 or 2.[12]

The second type of genetic variability is quasispecies, which are minor differences in HCV that are found in any individual. Quasispecies differ by less than 5 percent of their nucleotide sequence, but if you are infected with HCV, you may have as many as fifty slightly different viruses. The existence of these minor differences has major consequences:

- Although your body makes antibodies against HCV, these antibodies are often not effective against all of the quasispecies; because of this, the HCV persists and becomes chronic.
- Even if your body fights off the HCV, or you are successfully treated for it, you can easily become reinfected if you are exposed to the virus. The HCV antibodies that the body makes in response to HCV infection are not protective.
- Vaccines have not been effective because the antibodies they generate will not be active against all quasispecies.

CLINICAL FEATURES OF HCV INFECTION

In most people, HCV infection is silent; that is, there are no symptoms or symptoms are so minor that they do not prompt medical attention. A small number of patients with HCV have acute hepatitis, an obvious illness with symptoms such as flu-like symptoms, malaise, abdominal pain, dark urine, and jaundice. Liver enzymes can be high (ten to fifteen times the upper limit of normal). Acute hepatitis with high liver enzymes and even jaundice may not be associated with other symptoms and can go undetected. The symptoms usually resolve between two weeks and two months.

The majority (60–80 percent) of patients infected with HCV will develop chronic infection and persistently test positive for HCV antibody and HCV-RNA. Liver enzymes may be normal or modestly elevated (up to two times the upper limit of normal), and the levels often fluctuate. The levels of liver

---

TESTS COMMONLY USED IN THE INITIAL
EVALUATION OF PATIENTS WITH HCV INFECTION

- Liver enzymes (also referred to as liver function tests, but they measure liver injury not liver function).
- HCV antibody—detects exposure to HCV but not necessarily active infection. It remains positive after resolution or successful treatment of HCV.
- HCV-RNA—measures the number of virus particles in the blood. If positive, it denotes active infection. Often referred to as *viral load*.
- HCV genotype.
- Ultrasound—an imaging procedure that uses sound waves. It can detect nodularity of the liver that is characteristic of cirrhosis, and various types of cysts and tumors in the liver. It is used to screen patients with chronic HCV infection for liver cancer.

---

enzyme elevation do not correlate with the degree of liver damage, and you can have significant liver damage despite normal enzyme levels. Some patients clear the virus within the first three months of exposure: liver enzyme levels become normal and HCV-RNA undetectable, although HCV antibody remains detectable.

The lack of symptoms explains why so many people with HCV do not know that they have it. HCV is often discovered when you go to the doctor for some other reason, and a routine panel of blood tests, including liver enzymes, is ordered. If your enzymes are elevated, the next test is usually a hepatitis panel that includes HCV antibody. At that point, you may be referred to a gastroenterologist or hepatologist (liver specialist) for further evaluation and treatment.

If you have chronic HCV infection, your immune system keeps on trying, albeit unsuccessfully, to destroy the virus. **This immune response, rather than the virus itself, is what causes damage to the liver.** There are two main results of this immune attack within the liver: inflammation and fibrosis. In simple terms, inflammation is a response of the body to injury or infection that intends to destroy or isolate the underlying infectious agent or the damaged tissue. At the site of inflammation, there is an accumulation of white blood cells and other cells, and output of specialized molecules that further increase the reaction. Fibrosis is the body's attempt to heal by producing scar tissue, though it is the fibrosis that leads to most of the complications of HCV infection. Fibrosis can constrict the liver cells and interfere with their function. If the fibrosis is extensive and forms nodules, it is known as cirrhosis (see chapter 18, "Cirrhosis and the Spectrum of Liver Disease"). Cirrhosis can lead to serious complications, the need for liver transplantation, and death. HCV-associated cirrhosis is the most common cause for transplantation of the liver in the United States and other Western countries.[13]

Both of these processes, inflammation and fibrosis, can be viewed on a biopsy of the liver.

TESTS FOR LIVER FIBROSIS

- Liver biopsy—this is the standard test that has been used for decades. In addition to detecting fibrosis, it can assess inflammatory activity in HCV and can provide information that is not available any other way on the cause of liver disease. Liver biopsy is invasive: a needle is inserted into the liver under sterile conditions, and liver tissue is suctioned out. The tissue is stained and viewed under a microscope. There is a small risk of bleeding that can be serious. Also, there can be a sampling error: the tiny portion of the liver removed by the biopsy needle is usually but not always representative.
- Elastography—a non-invasive test that measures liver stiffness by measuring the speed of a low-frequency vibration traveling within the liver. Liver stiffness correlates with fibrosis, although other factors such as congestion and severe inflammation can increase stiffness of the liver. Elastography is not widely available outside of large hospital centers.
- Laboratory panels (APRI, FIB-4, FibroSURE, HepaScore)—these use a combination of blood tests that correlate with fibrosis. They are widely available and improving in accuracy.

Liver biopsies in HCV patients are staged for fibrosis, most commonly using the METAVIR system, which has stages F0–4.[14] Elastography and laboratory panels estimate the same fibrosis stages. The stages are as follows:

- F0—Chronic hepatitis with no fibrosis (scar tissue).
- F1—Portal fibrosis: fibrosis that is focused at the portal areas in the liver (areas in the liver where a portal vein, hepatic artery, and bile duct are seen in close proximity).
- F2—Portal fibrosis with visible fibrosis extending out from the portal area into the vast array of liver cells and tissue surrounding each portal area.
- F3—Portal fibrosis with thicker bands of fibrosis, including those which extend from one portal area to another.
- F4—Cirrhosis. There is extensive fibrosis of the liver, nodule formation, and distortion of the arrangement of the remaining liver cells.

Stage F3 has a significant risk of progressing to cirrhosis; stage F4 **is** cirrhosis and can progress to complications and liver failure (see chapter 18). There is widespread agreement that patients with F3–4 should be treated for HCV as soon as possible. Other stages can and should be treated.

HCV infection progresses very slowly, but after twenty to thirty years, about 5–20 percent will progress to cirrhosis. Alcohol increases the rate of fibrosis, as does male gender, obesity, insulin resistance, diabetes mellitus, and contracting HCV infection after age fifty.[15] In addition, HCV infection predisposes to primary liver cancer, also known as hepatocellular carcinoma, a cancer with a very poor prognosis. HCV infection increases the risk of hepatocellular carcinoma fifteen- to twenty-fold. HCV-associated hepatocellular carcinoma is the most rapidly increasing cause of cancer death in the United States, having tripled from 1990 to 2010, and is expected to keep increasing into the 2020s.[16] The death rate from all causes is also increased in chronic HCV infection.

"I HAVE HEPATITIS C. WHAT CAN I DO TO PREVENT IT FROM GETTING WORSE?"

- Exercise total abstinence from alcohol (most important).
- Lose weight if you are overweight.
- Eat a healthy, well-balanced diet, with emphasis on fruits, vegetables, and whole grains (see chapter 19, "Healthy Eating").
- Get enough exercise.
- Get vaccinated for hepatitis A and B if you are susceptible. You don't need another liver disease.
- Treat hepatitis B or HIV if present.

TREATMENT OF HCV INFECTION—OVERVIEW

Given the serious consequences of HCV infection, the medical profession considers treatment of this disorder to be a very high priority. Effective treatment of HCV infection stops the progression to cirrhosis, reduces the risk of hepatocellular carcinoma, and reduces the death rate from all causes. It may reverse cirrhosis in some cases. With each person treated, the spread of HCV infection becomes less likely.

In late 2013, a major step forward took place in HCV treatment with the approval of sofosbuvir (Sovaldi), one of a growing group of direct-acting antiviral drugs that were designed specifically to disrupt the HCV.

Direct-acting antivirals are highly effective and well tolerated. For example, in a study of treatment with the combination of ledipasvir and sofosbuvir (Harvoni) in previously untreated patients with HCV genotype 1, with or without cirrhosis, the response rate was 99 percent, and no patient had to stop the treatment because of side effects.[17] Direct-acting antivirals may have interactions with other drugs.

Before the release of sofosbuvir, all treatment regimens contained interferon, an injectable medication with many side effects, including flu-like symptoms, decreases in white blood cell and platelet counts, and potentially severe mental status changes (suicidal thoughts, completed suicides, and psychosis). Interferon was combined with ribavirin, an oral drug that causes anemia and other side effects (see box). At this time, interferon is almost never used in Western countries for treatment of HCV. Both interferon and ribavirin have antiviral effects that, unlike those of the direct-acting antivirals, are not specific for HCV. There now are several combination regimens of direct-acting antivirals, with or without ribavirin, and more are expected.

NOTES ON RIBAVIRIN

- Not a direct-acting antiviral, but has antiviral activity.
- Dosing of ribavirin is based on body weight.
- Ribavirin frequently causes anemia, which can be severe. Transfusions may be needed. Dose reduction of ribavirin may alleviate the anemia without compromising the effectiveness of the antiviral therapy.
- Other ribavirin side effects include rash, cough, jaundice, visual changes, and itching.
- Must not be used during pregnancy as it can cause birth defects. Pregnancy is not recommended for six months after stopping ribavirin.
- Men should not father children while taking ribavirin and for six months after the end of treatment.
- Two forms of contraception are recommended for a couple when one of them is taking ribavirin.
- Check for drug interactions.

The American Association for the Study of Liver Diseases (AASLD) and the Infectious Diseases Society of America (IDSA) jointly publish a web-based guidance statement on HCV that is frequently updated to provide clinicians with accurate, timely, and unbiased information on the best treatments for various groups of patients with HCV.[18] The AASLD-IDSA guidance states that all patients with HCV should be treated with the best available antiviral regimens unless they have a short life expectancy (less than one year) due to a non-liver-related condition. Furthermore, there is evidence that treating HCV at an earlier fibrosis stage (F0–2) is more beneficial than waiting for the patient to enter more advanced stages (F3–4). The guidance statement does not advise excluding drug users (including injection drug users) from treatment and opposes drug and alcohol screening.[19]

This recommendation of nearly universal treatment of HCV infection is not a reality due to the high cost of the medication. For example, sofosbuvir (Sovaldi) has a retail cost of $1,000 per pill and is used daily in combination with at least one other drug for eight, twelve, or less commonly twenty-four weeks; the combination pill ledipasvir and sofosbuvir (Harvoni), taken alone once a day for similar durations, lists at $1,125. Most insurance companies receive discounts of 40–75 percent. Some other direct-acting antivirals are only slightly less pricey, although the recently approved combination of elbasvir and grazoprevir (ZEPATIER) costs less (approximately $647 per pill).[20] The most common restriction imposed by insurance companies is limiting treatment to stages F3–4. Other restrictions include a required urine drug or alcohol screening, abstinence from alcohol and all illicit substances, must be in treatment (if HIV-positive) and in some cases have suppressed HIV viral load, and the prescriber must be in certain specialties.[21,22] In a 2015 analysis, thirty-three state Medicaid programs had policies that approved HCV treatment with direct-acting antivirals only for patients with stages F3–4 and denied such treatment to those with stages F0–2.[23]

There has been some pushback recently on both restricted access and the high prices of the new HCV drugs. In late 2015, the Centers for Medicare and Medicaid Services advised state Medicaid directors that they are required under federal law to cover effective HCV treatments.[24] A United States Sen-

MY EXPERIENCE WITH HCV TREATMENT IN MEDICAID PATIENTS

Many patients with HCV infection have Medicaid. For almost all of those that I see, I have been unable to secure coverage for direct-acting antivirals, even in patients with cirrhosis. I have encountered the following barriers:

- Must have fibrosis stage F3–4
- Must have fibrosis documented by liver biopsy, which is risky in advanced cirrhosis, or by elastography, which is not locally available
- Must have multiple urine drug screens negative for all drugs and alcohol
- Must have completed the six-month vaccination series for hepatitis B virus infection
- Constantly changing requirements with no prior notice

ate Finance Committee report has criticized the pricing of sofosbuvir and asserted that the price was based on maximizing profit rather than the actual costs of drug development and clinical trials.[25]

It is possible that the prices of direct-acting antivirals for HCV will go down as more drugs become available, and that access to these effective, life-saving drugs will increase. Treatment of HCV infection is cost-effective even in those with early stage fibrosis at the discounted rates most insurers, including Medicaid and the Veterans Administration, are getting.[26] Insurance and pharmaceutical companies can do more to ensure that the health of the public is safeguarded.

TREATMENT OF HCV INFECTION—THE DETAILS

The goal of treatment is to cure the HCV infection. You are considered cured if you achieve SVR12 (sustained virologic response twelve weeks after stopping treatment), meaning your HCV-RNA is undetectable, or negative, twelve weeks after the end of treatment. Additional goals of treatment are to reduce inflammation in the liver, stop the formation of fibrosis, and to reduce the risk of hepatocellular carcinoma.

Direct-acting antivirals for HCV infection are prescribed as a combination of at least two medicines that work on different parts of the virus. Doing so is necessary to achieve high cure rates and to reduce the odds of the HCV becoming resistant. Selecting the best antiviral drug combination is complex because the effectiveness is influenced by several factors:

- HCV genotype.
- Presence of cirrhosis, and whether the cirrhosis is compensated or decompensated (see chapter 18).
- History of prior antiviral therapy, and which drugs were used.
- HCV-RNA level.
- Resistance-associated variants. There are naturally occurring genetic variations in the HCV that render the virus more resistant to antiviral treatment with certain regimens (see discussion in the box).
- HIV infection.
- Side effects of the drugs.
- Drug interactions.

In addition, the availability of new drugs or new knowledge about existing drugs may factor into the decision making. In the future, the choice of antiviral drug may be individualized, based on the previous factors and new ones, as part of the trend toward personalized medicine that is seen in many areas of medical practice. Alternatively, medications that are active against all HCV genotypes in patients with all fibrosis stages could become the most widely used. This would allow more widespread treatment in countries where genotype and cirrhosis cannot be determined. On June 28, 2016, the U.S. Food and Drug Administration approved the combination of sofosbuvir and velpatasvir (Epclusa), which is effective against genotypes 1–6 and can be used in cirrhosis, though ribavirin should be added for moderate to severe cirrhosis.[27] Insurance companies may choose to cover only certain direct-acting antivirals.

While it is beyond the scope of this book to provide the recommendations for all subsets of patients, a few generalizations about treatment can be made. Response rates are lower in patients with cirrhosis, especially if they have been treated previously. Longer treatment may overcome some of this decreased responsiveness. Treatment duration ranges from eight to twenty-four weeks. Ribavirin is still needed in several subsets of patients.

VIRAL RESISTANCE AND POLYMORPHISMS

One new consideration with direct-acting antivirals for HCV is the possibility that the virus may become resistant to the treatment. This is uncommon now but could become more common in the future. Prevention of resistance is one of the reasons why direct-acting antivirals are given in combination and never as single agents, and why taking your HCV medication every day without interruption is so important. Polymorphisms, or genetic variations in the HCV, may occur naturally and can influence treatment. Polymorphisms in HCV are a result of small changes in the amino acid sequence of one of the viral proteins.

Little is known regarding the safety of direct-acting antivirals during pregnancy. Pregnancy testing should be done before any antiviral treatment for HCV is considered.

Once your physician has selected the best combination for you, the prescription will usually be sent to a specialty pharmacy that handles HCV treatment. The specialty pharmacy will request some information, such as genotype, fibrosis stage, and HCV-RNA level to confirm that the regimen is appropriate. It will then contact your insurance company, negotiate if necessary, obtain approval, and ship the medication directly to you. Before starting HCV treatment, you should discuss the possible side effects and drug interactions with your physician. There are drug interactions between antiviral

---

**DO NOT TAKE YOUR ANTIVIRAL
MEDICATION OVER THE SINK!**

You won't find this advice in guidelines or package inserts, but it is very important. How would you like to see your $1,000 pill circling the drain, just out of reach? It is very unlikely that you will get a replacement.

---

medications and many other medications, including common ones such as statins, proton pump inhibitors (see chapter 14, "Heartburn and Reflux"), and antacids. Make note of the date that you start treatment, as your physician will need this, and be sure to take your medication every day.

If you are hospitalized during your HCV treatment, bring your antiviral medication with you. Ask the hospital physician to contact the physician who prescribes your HCV treatment and discuss your continuing this medicine in the hospital. It is important not to interrupt antiviral therapy unless absolutely necessary.

After treatment, the key test is the HCV-RNA level twelve weeks after the end of treatment. If this is undetectable, you are cured! Repeating the HCV-RNA one more time in six to twelve months is a good idea, but further HCV-RNA testing is not needed assuming that there are not ongoing HCV risk factors. Other follow-up depends on the fibrosis stage. For stages F3–4, ultrasound and liver enzyme tests are recommended every six months to screen for hepatocellular carcinoma and should be continued for at least ten years. An EGD to screen for esophageal varices (see chapter 18) is advisable, with follow-up EGDs if varices are found. For stages F0–2, if you have no detectable HCV-RNA, no ongoing HCV risk factors, and no other liver disease (including fatty liver, with or without alcohol), you are now a regular patient like anyone who never had HCV infection![28]

THINKING OUTSIDE THE BOX ON PREVENTING HCV INFECTION

Most new cases of HCV infection are a result of injection drug use, and the United States is currently experiencing an epidemic of heroin use, much of which is by injection. The death rate attributed to heroin almost tripled from 2010 to 2013.[29] Because of this, a major increase in the incidence of HCV infection, affecting mainly young adults, is observed. Opioid dependence can be effectively treated in a physician's office using buprenorphine-naloxone, a long-acting opioid. A licensed physician can obtain a waiver to prescribe buprenorphine-naloxone for opioid dependence by completing an eight-hour course and having the capability of making referrals for counseling services. The need for physicians to provide this service greatly exceeds the availability,[30] and those physicians who treat HCV are in a good position to do so. I have provided opioid addiction treatment in my office since 2015. If more physicians did so, many cases of HCV infection could be prevented.

CASE REPORT—NEVER GIVE UP

Joline, a thirty-year-old female, came to the office in 1998 for evaluation of chronic hepatitis C. She had a history of surgery for a bleeding ulcer as a teenager, linked to heavy aspirin use for headaches. She received several blood transfusions at that time, which was before the discovery of hepatitis C (and hepatitis C testing of units of blood for transfusion). There was no history of injection drug use or alcohol use. Liver enzymes were elevated, HCV-RNA was 500,000 international units per milliliter (IU/ml), and liver biopsy showed moderate inflammatory activity and stage 3 liver fibrosis. The HCV genotype was 1a. She was treated with interferon and ribavirin, the standard treatment at that time. Although this treatment has many potential side effects, including flu-like symptoms and depression, she tolerated it well. Her HCV-RNA was negative at the end of treatment but was positive at 215,000 IU/ml six months later.

Three years later, she was treated with a peginterferon, a new version of interferon that was more effective, and ribavirin. She had increased fatigue during the treatment and cough attributed to ribavirin. HCV-RNA became negative during treatment, but she was found to have relapsed again when tested six months later.

She was reevaluated six years later and was found to have cirrhosis of the liver. She had an enlarged spleen and a very low platelet count (platelets are a blood cell that stops bleeding; an enlarged spleen may filter them excessively, resulting in low counts). EGD showed esophageal varices, and she was treated with a betablocker. Her condition gradually deteriorated over the next several years. She had episodes of esophageal variceal bleeding that were treated with variceal ligation and platelet transfusions. She was referred to a liver transplant center for evaluation, but her MELD score was too low to have a chance of receiving a new liver.

Thirteen years after her initial visit, a new antiviral regimen was approved by the FDA and became available: peginterferon, ribavirin, and telaprevir, the latter drug being one of the first two direct-acting antivirals (neither are in use in the United States today). Her platelet count had decreased to such low levels that the treatment was high risk. Since there was no significant option for liver transplantation, after an informed discussion she elected to try the new treatment. A new drug to boost platelets was not FDA approved but became available on a "compassionate use" basis.

Joline had a very rocky course with this treatment. She had fatigue, nausea, diarrhea, and loss of appetite. She became too weak to work. HCV-RNA became negative after four weeks of treatment, a response that is associated with excellent odds of success. Her anemia became severe, and red blood cell transfusions were needed on several occasions. The HCV-RNA remained negative during and at the end of treatment, but once again she relapsed.

Three years later, in 2014, she was treated with sofosbuvir and ribavirin, the first FDA-approved all-oral antiviral regimen for chronic hepatitis C. She had no significant side effects from the treatment and remained HCV-RNA negative after completion of treatment. She continues to be followed for cirrhosis, esophageal varices, enlarged spleen, and low platelet count, but she has remained stable and has not been hospitalized.

TAKE-HOME MESSAGES

- Anyone born from 1945 to 1965 should be tested for HCV. This test is covered by Medicare.
- Injection drug use causes most cases of HCV. If you ever injected drugs, even once, many years ago, you should be tested for HCV.
- If you have HCV, do not share a razor, toothbrush, or other implements that could cause minor bleeding.
- HCV has seven major strains, or genotypes. It also has multiple forms with minor differences that coexist within each patient, and this feature has prevented the creation of an HCV vaccine, at least so far.
- Most people have no symptoms at the time they acquire HCV. For this reason, the majority of people with HCV do not know that they have it.

- Important tests for HCV include HCV-RNA (often referred to as the viral load), which is the number of virus particles in the blood, and tests for liver fibrosis, or scar tissue.
- If you have HCV, do not drink any alcohol.
- The new drugs for HCV, known as direct-acting antivirals, are very effective, safe, and well tolerated, but very expensive. The high cost has resulted in the drugs being restricted by insurance companies to certain groups of patients; some call this rationing. The medical profession does not support these restrictions.
- The specific drugs recommended for HCV depend on many factors, most importantly genotype, the presence of cirrhosis, and any previous antiviral treatment. Ribavirin, an older drug that can cause severe anemia and birth defects, is needed for some patients.
- It is very important to take antiviral drugs every day as prescribed.

18

Cirrhosis and the Spectrum of Liver Disease

Cirrhosis of the liver is a condition in which there is extensive fibrosis, or scar tissue, in the liver. The fibrosis gradually constricts the liver cells and disrupts their function, potentially leading to serious complications, the need for liver transplantation, or death. Cirrhosis is estimated to be the twelfth leading cause of death in the United States,[1] but the incidence of cirrhosis and the death rate are expected to increase in this decade and beyond because of the aging of the baby boomers who acquired hepatitis C virus (HCV) infection in great numbers forty to fifty years earlier (see chapter 17, "Hepatitis C") and from the current epidemic of obesity and fatty liver disease (see below). Of note, the death rate from cirrhosis increased by 3 percent from 2012 to 2013.[2]

For years, it was thought that liver fibrosis was permanent and cirrhosis irreversible. However, data from studies of antiviral therapy of chronic HCV and hepatitis B virus infections have shown that cirrhosis can be reversed after successful antiviral treatment.[3] After stopping drinking, patients with alcoholic cirrhosis improve, sometimes dramatically, with resolution of complications, but reversal of cirrhosis in this setting is not expected. Nevertheless, there are benefits of stopping drinking at all stages of alcoholic liver disease, even the most advanced. If the underlying cause is not treated, cirrhosis will progress at varying rates.

CAUSES OF CIRRHOSIS

Although cirrhosis is commonly associated with extensive use of alcohol, there are many causes of cirrhosis. The three most common in the United States today are alcohol, chronic HCV infection, and non-alcoholic fatty liver disease. Fatty liver is common in alcoholic liver disease but is also seen in obesity without alcohol use, a problem that has increased greatly in the last twenty to thirty years. Table 18.1 shows the causes of cirrhosis, including those that are common in a hepatology (liver disease) practice. The following sections will review the most common entities.

Table 18.1. Causes of Cirrhosis

Common	Common in a Hepatology Practice	Less Common or Rare
• Alcohol • Chronic HCV infection • Non-alcoholic fatty liver disease	• Chronic hepatitis B infection • Hereditary hemochromatosis • Autoimmune hepatitis • Primary biliary cholangitis • Drug toxicity • Cryptogenic	• Wilson's disease • Alpha-1 antitrypsin deficiency • Congestive heart failure

ALCOHOLIC LIVER DISEASE

Alcoholic liver disease occurs in about 15 percent of long-term heavy drinkers. There is no definite safe limit of alcohol intake, but larger amounts and longer duration of alcohol increase the odds. Liver disease can occur with any type of alcoholic beverage, including beer. Women metabolize alcohol differently than men and develop liver disease after smaller quantities and shorter durations of alcohol intake. Malnutrition and chronic HCV infection can accelerate the course of alcoholic liver injury.[4,5]

Alcoholic cirrhosis is preceded by fatty liver disease in almost all patients and by alcoholic hepatitis in a few. Patients with alcoholic hepatitis are severely ill with fever, jaundice, abdominal pain, and elevated white cell counts. They may have esophageal varices with bleeding or ascites. Total abstinence from alcohol is essential for all stages of alcoholic liver disease. Alcohol counseling and self-help groups such as Alcoholics Anonymous are important. Naltrexone, an opioid blocker, can reduce the craving for alcohol. Hospitalized patients with alcoholic liver disease may develop symptoms of alcohol withdrawal, including tremors, seizures, and hallucinations because admission to the hospital brings alcohol intake to an abrupt halt. Alcohol withdrawal is a medical emergency and is treated with intravenous fluids, sedation, and close monitoring. Alcoholic hepatitis is treated with intravenous fluids, nutritional support, and acid blockers. Severe alcoholic hepatitis is also treated with corticosteroids, most commonly prednisolone.[6]

NON-ALCOHOLIC FATTY LIVER DISEASE

This disorder is increasing in frequency along with the worldwide epidemic of obesity and will soon be the most common cause of liver disease and cirrhosis. Approximately two billion adults worldwide are overweight and 600 million are obese.[7] The global prevalence of non-alcoholic fatty liver disease is 25 percent. Type 2 diabetes mellitus (see glossary), especially when not well controlled, is often a contributing factor. Non-alcoholic fatty liver disease is closely linked with obesity, elevated blood lipids (fats), hypertension, and type 2 diabetes, all of which are risk factors for heart disease, a major cause of death in people with non-alcoholic fatty liver disease.[8]

Some patients progress from simple fatty liver to non-alcoholic steatohepatitis (NASH), in which there is an inflammatory reaction in the liver in addition to fat deposits. Further progression of NASH may lead to liver fibrosis and cirrhosis, although the rate of such progression is slow. Nevertheless, given the enormous number of overweight and obese people, large increases in the frequency of cirrhosis, liver transplantation, and liver-related deaths from NASH are expected in the coming decades.

Most patients with non-alcoholic fatty liver disease have elevated liver enzymes on blood testing, but these can be normal. Treatment includes weight reduction, a healthy diet (see chapter 19, "Healthy Eating"), exercise, and avoidance of alcohol. Vitamin E supplementation is thought to be of some benefit for patients with NASH who do not have diabetes.

CHRONIC HEPATITIS B VIRUS INFECTION

Chronic hepatitis B virus infection is a major problem worldwide but is becoming uncommon in the United States due to the routine use of the hepatitis B vaccine during the last twenty-five years. Chronic hepatitis B in the United States is now mainly seen in immigrants. There are medications that can suppress the hepatitis B virus, including entecavir and tenofovir, which are the most common ones used. However, relapse is common when the drug is discontinued. Chronic hepatitis B virus infection is a major risk factor for hepatocellular carcinoma, and ongoing monitoring with ultrasound is necessary.

HEREDITARY HEMOCHROMATOSIS

This inherited disorder of iron metabolism is relatively common in Caucasian populations. The underlying defect is in the upper small intestine, where an excessive amount of iron is absorbed yet the area appears normal on routine tests, including EGD. The excess iron deposits are found in the liver, heart, pancreas, joints, and other organs. Most patients with hereditary hemochromatosis have no symptoms and are identified when a blood test shows an elevated level of iron or ferritin, the storage form of iron. It is possible that the disease may progress to cirrhosis or congestive heart failure without being recognized. Advanced cases are associated with diabetes, arthritis, or a bronze discoloration of the skin, all of which develop gradually.

Most cases of hereditary hemochromatosis are related to two major mutations in the HFE gene, the gene for hemochromatosis (HFE stands for high Fe, Fe being the chemical symbol for iron). Testing for the two major mutations is routinely available. Family members should be tested. If you have this disorder and have children, testing the other parent for iron levels and the HFE gene mutations is a quick way to assess your children's risk of developing the manifestations of this disease in the future. If the other parent tests negative, the children will not have the disease, since to get hemochromatosis one must inherit a mutation from each parent. Treatment is with phlebotomy, or removal of blood from the body. Phlebotomies are done weekly until the body is depleted of the excess iron, and then gradually reduced in frequency. In some patients the iron does not reaccumulate after prolonged phlebotomy treatment, and phlebotomies can be discontinued. Early treatment can prevent cirrhosis and its complications.

AUTOIMMUNE HEPATITIS

This type of hepatitis is not related to a virus or any other infection. The term hepatitis actually means inflammation of the liver from any cause. Autoimmune hepatitis is a disorder in which your immune system detects something on the surface of the liver cell that it does not recognize and tries to reject it. The onset of the disease may be gradual or abrupt, ranging from no symptoms or mild fatigue to the sudden onset of abdominal pain or jaundice. Autoimmune hepatitis is more common in females. Laboratory tests usually show autoantibodies, or antibodies against normal cell components. Liver biopsy is helpful in establishing the diagnosis, and an accurate diagnosis is important because of the need for long-term medications.

Treatment is initially with corticosteroids such as prednisone, which suppresses the immune response and leads to rapid improvement in most. After you respond to prednisone, the dose is reduced and azathioprine can be added to maintain remission. It is very important not to stop treatment on your own, as this can lead to a relapse, which may be more severe than the original presentation. Many patients eventually can be maintained on azathioprine alone, and all treatment can be stopped in some.

Side effects of prednisone and azathioprine are reviewed in chapter 10, "Crohn's Disease and Ulcerative Colitis (Inflammatory Bowel Disease)."

PRIMARY BILIARY CHOLANGITIS
(PREVIOUSLY PRIMARY BILIARY CIRRHOSIS)

In primary biliary cholangitis, the focus of inflammation is the small bile ducts within the liver. It is thought to be an autoimmune disease, but the cause is unknown. Itching, which can be severe, and jaundice are common symptoms. Primary biliary cholangitis is much more common in middle-aged women. As in autoimmune hepatitis, autoantibodies are usually present and can help in the diagnosis. Primary biliary cholangitis may overlap with autoimmune hepatitis. Treatment with ursodeoxycholic acid, a naturally occurring bile acid, can improve liver test results and significantly slow the progression of the disease. Jaundice can be seen with advanced disease, and liver transplantation may be the only life-saving treatment. The itching can be treated with several medications: antihistamines; cholestyramine, a drug that binds bile salts; and naltrexone, an opioid antagonist. Patients with primary biliary cholangitis often have bone disease that should be treated if present.

In May 2016, the Food and Drug Administration (FDA) approved obeticholic acid for treatment of primary biliary cholangitis.[9] Obeticholic acid lowers liver test results and can be used alone or with ursodeoxycholic acid.[10]

The name of this disease has been changed from *primary biliary cirrhosis*,[11] because although it may progress to cirrhosis, it does not always do so.

PRIMARY SCLEROSING CHOLANGITIS

This disorder, also of unknown cause, is strongly associated with ulcerative colitis (see chapter 10, "Crohn's Disease and Ulcerative Colitis [Inflammatory Bowel Disease]"). Most patients with primary sclerosing cholangitis have ulcerative colitis; some do not have inflammatory bowel disease, and a few have Crohn's disease. Most patients with inflammatory bowel disease do not have primary sclerosing cholangitis, however. Primary sclerosing cholangitis is most common in young adult males. It can involve the entire biliary system. Symptoms include fatigue, itching, and trouble absorbing fat, including fat-soluble vitamins. Like primary biliary cholangitis, this disorder may overlap with autoimmune hepatitis. It is diagnosed with MRCP or ERCP (see chapter 16, "Gallbladder and Pancreas"), which show areas of narrowing and dilation leading to a beaded appearance of the bile ducts. There is no effective medication. Liver transplantation is appropriate for advanced cases. There is an increased incidence of cholangiocarcinoma, a cancer of the bile ducts with a very poor prognosis, in primary sclerosing cholangitis.

DRUG-INDUCED LIVER DISEASE

A huge number of drugs and chemicals can cause liver injury, but relatively few cause or contribute to cirrhosis. Methotrexate, used for rheumatoid arthritis (and rarely for inflammatory bowel disease), and nitrofurantoin, for urinary tract infections, may lead to cirrhosis. Antibiotics are the most common cause of acute liver injury, and increasing numbers of cases are seen in herbal and dietary supplements (see chapter 19, "Healthy Eating").

A common question is whether people with liver disease can take acetaminophen safely. The main problem with acetaminophen is overdose, which can lead to acute, severe liver failure. Overdose of acetaminophen can be accidental (unintentional), in which a person keeps taking it for headaches, back pain, or some other painful condition without keeping track of how much they are taking. This problem is compounded by the fact that acetaminophen is an ingredient in many over-the-counter pain relievers as well as the most commonly prescribed opioid pain relievers, including codeine, hydrocodone, and oxycodone. If you take acetaminophen plus a variety of other pain medications every few hours, it is possible to reach a toxic level of acetaminophen without realizing it. Acetaminophen is also used for suicide attempts (intentional overdose).

Acetaminophen is metabolized by both a major and minor pathway, and the minor pathway results in production of a toxic metabolite (breakdown product). Normally, the toxic metabolite is rendered harmless by binding to a substance called glutathione, but if either too much acetaminophen is taken or if glutathione is depleted, the toxic metabolite cannot be inactivated and will bind to liver cells. Such binding causes cell necrosis and death. Liver transplantation can be life-saving.

Chronic use of alcohol activates the liver enzymes involved in the minor pathway. Even standard doses of acetaminophen can cause toxicity in long-term alcohol users.

If you have non-alcoholic liver disease, including cirrhosis, you may take acetaminophen safely. It is best to take the smallest dose possible and for the shortest duration. This should be discussed with your personal physician. Acetaminophen is the safest non-prescription pain regimen for most people with non-alcoholic liver disease,[12] and non-steroidal anti-inflammatory drugs such as ibuprofen are more risky (may cause fluid retention and gastrointestinal bleeding). Patients with past or present chronic alcoholism should avoid acetaminophen or take minimal doses. For patients with cirrhosis, a maximum of 2 grams per day has been suggested.[13] A limit of 8 grams per week, indicating that one should not take 2 grams every day, is reasonable. Glutathione can become depleted in advanced cirrhosis, fasting, malnutrition, or illnesses in which there is poor oral intake, and standard doses of acetaminophen can cause toxicity in these situations as well.[14]

CRYPTOGENIC CIRRHOSIS

This refers to cirrhosis of unknown cause. Fatty liver disease with normal liver enzyme tests may account for many of these cases.

WILSON'S DISEASE

Wilson's disease is a very rare but treatable genetic disease of copper metabolism that can cause cirrhosis. Too much copper accumulates in the liver and other organs. It is most commonly seen in adolescents or young adults and can be associated with abnormal body movements or psychiatric disorders. The treatment includes compounds that bind the copper, thus lowering the high levels in the body.

ALPHA-1 ANTITRYPSIN DEFICIENCY

This is an inherited liver disease that can be diagnosed at any age. It can be seen in family members. Genetic tests are routinely available. It can be associated with lung disease, along with the liver disease. It often comes to light during evaluation of cirrhosis, and liver biopsy can provide confirmatory information. Infusions of alpha-1 antitrypsin are beneficial for the lung but not liver manifestations. Liver transplantation is the definitive treatment for advanced cirrhosis secondary to alpha-1 antitrypsin deficiency.

CONGESTIVE HEART FAILURE

When the heart cannot pump out enough blood, the blood trying to get to the heart will back up and lead to congestion of the liver. If this process is chronic, cirrhosis can develop, sometimes referred to as cardiac cirrhosis. Cardiac cirrhosis is seen less often these days because of better treatment of heart disease.

COMPENSATED AND DECOMPENSATED CIRRHOSIS

An important distinction in cirrhosis is whether it is compensated or decompensated. In compensated cirrhosis, patients generally feel well and do not have severe abnormalities on laboratory testing. Such patients may remain stable for years. Decompensated cirrhosis denotes the appearance of complications, the most common of which are esophageal varices, ascites, and hepatic encephalopathy. Patients with decompensated cirrhosis look and feel chronically ill and have reduced survival based on the severity of complications. Liver transplantation is usually considered.

PORTAL HYPERTENSION

All organs have arteries that bring in blood containing oxygen and veins that return the blood toward the heart after oxygen removal. The liver is unusual in that it has a dual blood supply. It has the hepatic artery, which brings in blood carrying oxygen, but this is only 25 percent of the incoming blood flow. The other 75 percent comes from the portal vein, which is the convergence of veins leaving the small intestine, stomach, spleen, and pancreas. The portal vein and the veins that feed into it are collectively known as the portal venous system. A major function of the portal venous system is the transporting of food particles that are absorbed in the small intestine. These nutrients are brought to the liver for processing and distribution.

When cirrhosis is present, the blood entering the portal venous system meets increased resistance because of the fibrosis in the liver, and the blood pressure in this system goes up. If the pressure becomes high enough, the blood will reverse its course and follow the path of least resistance, which usually means backing up into the veins of the esophagus, stomach, spleen, and rectum. These veins can become engorged and swollen and are known as varices (the singular is varix). In some patients, the portal pressure becomes so high that the veins, especially those of the esophagus, can rupture and cause a massive, life-threatening bleed. The blood may be vomited or may pass through the GI tract, resulting in melena (see chapter 13, "Evaluation of the Esophagus, Stomach, and Small Intestine"). The increased portal pressure, also referred to as portal hypertension, contributes to the development of ascites as well.

Cirrhosis is the most common cause of portal hypertension, but there are others, such as a large blood clot in the portal vein.

ESOPHAGEAL VARICES

The best way to diagnose esophageal varices is with an EGD, during which varices are easily visible (figure 18.1).

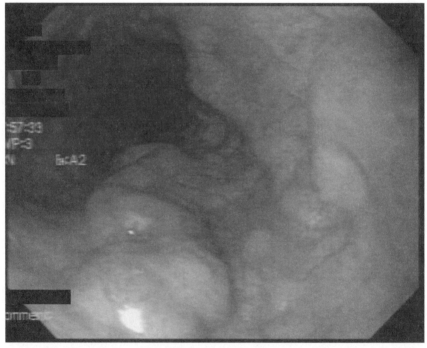

Figure 18.1. Esophageal varices: dilated veins seen in the esophagus during an EGD.
Source: David M. Novick, *Esophageal Varices,* July 2016.

It is standard practice to do an EGD when cirrhosis is diagnosed to assess for varices. If they are detected before they have bled, preventive measures can be initiated. Certain medications, nadolol and propranolol (known as non-selective beta blockers), can reduce the portal pressure and consequently the risk of bleeding. They can also be used to reduce the risk of a subsequent bleed in patients who have had an episode of variceal hemorrhage.

Larger varices can be treated with esophageal variceal ligation. In this technique, an adapter fitted with rubber bands is placed onto the tip of the scope, following which the scope is advanced into the esophagus. A varix is suctioned into the adapter, and a rubber band is then deployed onto the varix. This can be repeated several times. A clot will form in the part of the varix that is pinched off, by the rubber band, and eventually the clot and the rubber band will fall off leaving an ulcer that then heals with scar tissue. This procedure is repeated at intervals until the varices are obliterated.

Esophageal variceal ligation can also be used to treat actively bleeding varices. Variceal bleeding can be massive, and stopping the bleeding is a life-saving procedure that will invariably be done at the hospital. The management of variceal bleeding can be extremely complex and includes medications that decrease portal blood flow, antibiotics, fluids, protecting the airway from vomited blood, and additional procedures if bleeding cannot be controlled. For massive bleeding not controlled by variceal ligation, the next step is often a transjugular intrahepatic portosystemic shunt, or TIPS. Performed by interventional radiologists, a TIPS is a hollow device, or stent, that is placed in a way that connects a branch of the portal vein with a branch of the hepatic vein. Blood will flow more easily from the portal vein through the stent, resulting in decreased portal pressure and cessation of the bleeding. Expert medical judgment is required, as there are many potential limitations and complications of the TIPS procedure.

ASCITES

Ascites is the abnormal accumulation of fluid in the abdominal cavity. It is the most common complication of cirrhosis, and more than 80 percent of cases of ascites are a result of cirrhosis.[15] Other causes of ascites include cancer, congestive heart failure, tuberculosis, pancreatitis, and obstruction of the veins through which blood exits the liver.

Ascites can become massive, although it usually develops gradually. Someone affected with ascites may have obvious abdominal distention, and the abdomen may contain more than twenty liters of fluid. Ascites is often accompanied by swelling of the ankles or legs (edema), and in some cases by muscle wasting.

Ascites is an indicator that the cirrhosis is decompensated and associated with a poor prognosis. Less than half of patients with cirrhosis who develop ascites will survive five years.[16]

When ascites is diagnosed, it is important that a paracentesis (abdominal tap), or withdrawal of fluid from the abdominal cavity for testing, be performed. Ultrasound is usually used to guide the needle. The fluid is tested for infection and examined for cancer cells. Also, determining the level of albumin (a protein) in the ascites and comparing it to the level in the blood can strongly suggest whether the ascites is a result of portal hypertension or another cause.

Treatment of ascites consists of the following:

- Treat the underlying cause. If alcohol is a factor, total abstinence is essential.
- Low-sodium (salt) diet. A sodium intake of less than 2 grams per day is recommended. This needs to be done rigorously by reading food labels, not just avoiding added salt (see chapter 19). Avoid canned or processed foods, and do not eat in restaurants. Avoid salt substitutes as many contain potassium. Working with a dietician can be helpful.
- Diuretics (commonly referred to as water pills)—these are medications that increase the excretion of sodium and fluids through the kidneys and into the urine. For most patients with ascites resulting from cirrhosis, the drugs furosemide and spironolactone will be used, often in combination. These diuretics work on different parts of the kidney and complement each other. Your doctor will monitor your electrolytes (especially potassium) and kidney function when diuretics are used. A low-sodium diet is essential for diuretics to be effective.
- Measure your weight every morning after urinating, and keep a chart.
- Keep a food diary if you are not losing weight, and then review it for high-sodium foods.
- Fluid intake is not limited unless the sodium in the blood is low.

The effectiveness of diuretic therapy can be assessed by following the body weight. A loss of three to four pounds per week is reasonable, and loss of more than seven pounds per week is not recommended. If you are losing more than four pounds per week, let your physician know, as diuretics may need to be reduced. If weight loss does not occur with increasing doses of diuretics, either you are not following the low-sodium diet, or the ascites has become refractory. Refractory ascites has a very poor prognosis, with only a 50 percent survival at one year, and it warrants referral for liver transplantation in most cases.[17] The ascites will then be treated with large-volume paracentesis, often at regular intervals. TIPS is also an option for refractory ascites.

There are two additional complications that may occur in patients with cirrhosis and ascites: spontaneous bacterial peritonitis and hepatorenal syndrome. Spontaneous bacterial peritonitis is an infection of ascites fluid not caused by a surgically treatable source. It is a medical emergency that requires prompt diagnosis and treatment. Typical symptoms are abdominal pain, fever, or altered mental status in a patient with ascites. Such patients should go promptly to the ER, have a paracentesis for testing of the fluid, receive antibiotics as soon as possible after the paracentesis, and be admitted to the hospital. After treatment, prevention of recurrence is promoted by taking antibiotics once per week.

Hepatorenal syndrome is a decline in renal (kidney) function caused by the body's response to advanced portal hypertension in patients with ascites. Essentially, the blood vessels in the kidneys constrict in response to severe dilation of the blood vessels of the abdominal cavity and the general circulation, which in turn is a response to portal hypertension.[18] Hepatorenal syndrome is a functional renal failure, in that the kidneys do not function properly but exhibit no structural damage. Patients with hepatorenal syndrome are sick enough to be hospitalized and are treated with intravenous fluids, infusions of albumin (a protein that circulates in the blood), and medications that raise the blood pressure. Liver transplantation can be lifesaving but needs to be done relatively quickly as the prognosis of hepatorenal syndrome is otherwise poor.[19]

HEPATIC ENCEPHALOPATHY

This is the third major complication of cirrhosis, and it can coexist with esophageal varices and ascites. Hepatic encephalopathy is a spectrum of mental status changes in patients with cirrhosis. The changes may range from those so minimal that only a very close family member or friend would notice, to stupor, disorientation, and coma. One classification system (West Haven Criteria)[20] describes grades 1–4 as follows:

- Grade 1: Trivial lack of awareness, euphoria, anxiety, shortened attention span, and impaired performance of addition.
- Grade 2: Lethargy, apathy, minimal disorientation for time or place, subtle personality change, inappropriate behavior, and impaired performance of subtraction. Asterixis, a flapping tremor that is typical of hepatic encephalopathy, is usually present.
- Grade 3: Somnolence to semistupor. Confusion and gross disorientation, but responsive to verbal stimuli. Asterixis is present.
- Grade 4: Coma (unresponsive to verbal or noxious stimuli).

In addition to the grades of hepatic encephalopathy, this disorder is also divided into two levels of severity: covert and overt. They encompass the entire spectrum of mental status changes in cirrhosis and hepatic encephalopathy. Patients with cirrhosis but little or no impairment on routine clinical and laboratory evaluation may have abnormalities on tests of concentration, decision making, coordination, and reaction times.[21] Such patients are catego-rized as having covert hepatic encephalopathy, whereas clinically apparent hepatic encephalopathy, with disorientation, asterixis, or other manifestations of grades 2–4, is overt hepatic encephalopathy. Grade 1 hepatic encephalopa-thy is included in the covert group because its evaluation is very subjective.

At this time, there is no standard test for covert hepatic encephalopathy that is routinely available, accurate, and able to be administered by persons without special expertise.[22] A smartphone app, EncephalApp Stroop (released in 2016), may be a convenient screening test but needs further evaluation. Covert hepatic encephalopathy therefore often goes unrecognized, but it is associated with increased progression to overt hepatic encephalopathy and a higher rate of motor vehicle violations and accidents, and responds to treat-ment with the medications discussed on page 163.

DRIVING AND HEPATIC ENCEPHALOPATHY

A challenging issue in the management of hepatic encephalopathy is when driving privileges should be restricted. If you have cirrhosis and hepatic encephalopathy, your reflexes may not be quick enough to prevent an acci-dent, and you and others may be at risk if you drive. It is often necessary to restrict driving privileges, which to many people means a loss of freedom.

It is very important that the risks of motor vehicle use be discussed with patients with hepatic encephalopathy. In my experience, the best approach is to involve family members or close friends in the discussion. Offers to help with driving will often materialize. Poor performance in driving simulator studies predicts real-life accidents and traffic violations, and referral for a professional driving assessment may be appropriate.[23] As a last resort, the physician can report the patient to the Department of Motor Vehicles; even the threat to do so imparts the seriousness of the situation. Such reporting is not considered a violation of confidentiality.[24] State regulations may vary, and ultimately it is up to the state to determine whether or not someone may drive.

The underlying problem in hepatic encephalopathy is that the diseased liver can no longer process certain toxic substances that are absorbed from the intestinal tract. The best known of these and the one that is routinely measured is ammonia, but there are many others. These substances are not cleared by the liver, and therefore enter the circulation and reach the brain, where they cause the changes listed previously.

Hepatic encephalopathy is often triggered by a particular inciting event. The most recognized such events include the following:

- Infection
- Gastrointestinal bleeding
- Constipation
- Eating a large-protein meal (uncommon)
- Dehydration, including that caused by excessive use of diuretics
- Low potassium
- Medications that affect the brain, such as sedatives or opioid pain medications

Treatment of hepatic encephalopathy starts with identifying and correcting precipitating events. Then the treatment is with lactulose, a disaccharide that is not absorbed, makes the colon more acidic, and has a laxative effect. These effects can clear the toxins and improve the mental status. Lactulose may also alter the bowel bacteria in a favorable way. Lactulose is the primary drug that is used for hepatic encephalopathy, both as a treatment and a maintenance medication. Lactulose is effective and inexpensive but is the source of many complaints because of the very sweet taste and side effects of gas and diarrhea. The recommended dose of lactulose is that which leads to two to three soft stools per day, but it is not easy to get the maximum improvement in mental status with such limited adverse effects.

The other medication that is very effective in hepatic encephalopathy is rifaximin, a poorly absorbed antibiotic that is well tolerated[25] but limited by high cost. It works by decreasing the production of ammonia by gut bacteria.[26] Rifaximin is also used in irritable bowel syndrome (see chapter 9).

An older treatment for hepatic encephalopathy that is no longer recommended is protein restriction.[27] Patients with cirrhosis need protein and are at risk for loss of muscle protein. In the presence of cirrhosis, the liver can no longer store adequate amounts of glycogen, a storage form of glucose. Glucose is so critical for energy production by the body that if no other source is available it will break down muscle protein, and the amino acids that result will be chemically converted to glucose. This process is common in patients with advanced cirrhosis, many of whom have obvious muscle wasting. Therefore, patients with cirrhosis should **avoid fasting** and especially should have a **daily breakfast** and a **late-night snack**.[28] They should have **sufficient protein** in the diet, most of which should be **dairy or vegetable** protein.

MALNUTRITION

Malnutrition is common in cirrhosis and is a factor that can lead to decompensation. Malnutrition results from inadequate intake of food and poor absorption of nutrients.

The following nutritional interventions can be helpful in patients with cirrhosis:

- Do not restrict protein.
- Eat mostly vegetable and dairy protein when possible.
- Eat breakfast.
- Eat a late-night snack that includes carbohydrates.
- Include foods with antioxidants, such as coffee and dark chocolate.
- Take probiotics.
- When taking nutritional supplements, they should be enriched with branched-chain amino acids, which are a group of essential amino acids (see glossary) that become depleted in cirrhosis. Replacement of branched-chain amino acids may have beneficial effects in cirrhosis beyond improvement in nutritional status.[29] Discuss with your doctor or a nutritionist.
- Avoid raw shellfish, which may contain a bacteria (*Vibrio vulnificus*) that is dangerous in patients with cirrhosis.
- Frequent small meals in patients with massive ascites.

LIVER TRANSPLANTATION

If you have cirrhosis, liver transplantation can be life-saving, but the decision to refer for liver transplantation requires careful thought. The transplant center will require an extensive medical evaluation, in some cases duplicating tests that were done by your local gastroenterologist and other physicians. You will need to consider your tolerance for undergoing such testing as well as a long surgical procedure that has many potential complications, including death. You will need much support from family and friends, especially for transportation if you are too sick to drive yourself. If you have a history of drug or alcohol abuse, you will not be excluded from consideration for a liver transplant, but you are expected now to be totally abstinent. You may have to undergo drug or alcohol counseling even if the substance use was many years ago and you believe that you no longer have the problem. Once you are "listed" (placed on the waiting list) for transplantation, you may face a very long wait while grappling with ascites, encephalopathy, or other complications which can be extremely unpleasant. After transplantation, you will need to take medications with potentially severe toxicity in order to prevent your body from rejecting the new liver. It is wise to consider all of these issues and to discuss them with your family before proceeding with the evaluation for liver transplantation.

There are not enough livers to accommodate everyone who might benefit from a liver transplant. Every year, many people die while on the waiting list, and the families of many potential donors are too grief-stricken to think that their tragedy could save someone else's life. **If you are reading this, please consider becoming an organ donor and encourage others to do the same**.

Because of the shortage of livers for transplantation, a system has been devised to treat the sickest first. It may seem surprising that the rating system does not take into account the major complications discussed previously. This is because the management of these complications has greatly improved in the last several decades, and their presence is not an accurate predictor of survival. The system used is the MELD (Model of End-Stage Liver Disease) score, which uses a formula that depends on three common blood tests: serum bilirubin, serum creatinine, and prothrombin time. The MELD score correlates with survival. Online calculators are available. If small liver cancers are present that can be cured with transplantation, additional MELD points are given, and such cancers are usually treated while the patient awaits liver transplantation.

Liver transplantation is a potential treatment for many patients with cirrhosis and also those with severe acute liver failure from various causes including acetaminophen toxicity and the supplement-related liver injuries discussed in chapter 19. It is not done in patients with uncontrolled infection outside of the liver, most non-liver cancers, advanced heart or lung disease, or active alcohol or substance use. It is considered more carefully in patients over age seventy but can be done in some if they are otherwise healthy.

Most livers for transplantation are procured from people under age sixty who have died from head trauma. These cadaver donors must not have had infection, abdominal injury, or other types of medical instability. They may have had hepatitis B or C without significant liver injury if they are to be transplanted into recipients with those viruses. The donor and recipient must have compatible blood types.

CAN I DONATE PART OF MY LIVER?

Some liver transplant centers offer living donor liver transplantation, in which a healthy person has a portion of their liver surgically removed and immediately transplanted into the recipient. This procedure has several advantages, notably that the recipient need not wait until he or she has reached the most advanced stages of cirrhosis and is sick enough to have a sufficiently high MELD score to receive a transplant. The liver will regenerate in both the donor and recipient, resulting in normal liver function, assuming no complications occur.[30,31]

Living donor liver transplantation does involve risk to the donor, who should be in excellent health and will need to undergo an extensive medical and psychological evaluation. Such live donations must be entirely voluntary.

TAKE-HOME MESSAGES

- Cirrhosis of the liver is caused by extensive fibrosis, or scar tissue in the liver. It is the twelfth leading cause of death in the United States.
- There are many causes of cirrhosis besides alcohol. Chronic HCV infection and non-alcoholic fatty liver disease are the most common.
- There is no definite safe limit of alcohol consumption. Although many heavy drinkers never develop cirrhosis, a greater volume of alcohol consumed and a longer duration of drinking will increase the odds.
- Beer contains alcohol and if ingested in sufficient quantities can cause all stages of alcoholic liver injury, including cirrhosis.
- Women develop alcoholic liver disease with smaller volumes of alcohol than men do.
- Non-alcoholic fatty liver disease is increasing with the current epidemic of obesity.
- Esophageal varices, ascites, and hepatic encephalopathy are serious complications that require urgent attention.
- Eating breakfast and having a late-night snack are important to reduce the occurrence of muscle breakdown in cirrhosis.

19

Healthy Eating

There is much good nutritional information available today. This chapter will give you the basic tools to make wise dietary choices. Recommended diets for various GI disorders will be found in their respective chapters. For maintaining health or weight loss, I will give general comments and recommendations without endorsing any particular diet. In fact, I don't like the term "diet," as it connotes struggle, quitting, and failure; I much prefer the concept of "Don't diet; eat healthy."

BACKGROUND INFORMATION ON FOOD

There are three main components of food: fat, carbohydrate, and protein. All are necessary, and healthy eating consists of finding the right balance. As a rough guideline, 25–35 percent of calories should come from fat, 15–25 percent from protein, and 40–55 percent from carbohydrates. Figure 19.1 shows the proportions of common food types that will meet this goal. The plate is intentionally small when compared to the fork.

In May 2016, the U.S. Food and Drug Administration (FDA) issued an updated version of the nutrition facts label that is required on foods that it regulates. Figure 19.2 shows the new label and the changes from the previous version. The number of calories per serving is larger and the serving size is in bold type. A section on added sugars has been added (see discussion under carbohydrates). Vitamin D and potassium amounts and percentages of the daily value based on a 2,000-calorie diet have been added, as many people do not get enough of these in their diet; vitamin A and C amounts and percentages are now optional. A footnote explaining the daily value has been added.

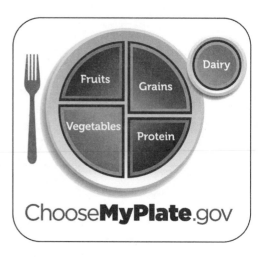

Figure 19.1. What your healthy plate should look like. Note the small portion sizes.

Source: U.S. Department of Agriculture, http://www .choosemyplate.gov/myplate-graphic-resources, United States Department of Agriculture (USDA). *Choose My Plate.* From the USDA Center for Nutrition Policy and Promotion's ChooseMyPlate .gov website.

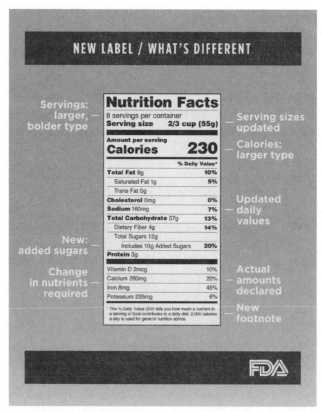

Figure 19.2. Nutrition label.

Source: U.S. Food and Drug Administration, http://www.fda.gov/Food/Guidance Regulation/GuidanceDocumentsRegulatoryInformation/LabelingNutrition/ ucm385663.htm, Food and Drug Administration. *New Label/What's Different.*

The FDA also changed the amount of food in a serving to more realistically reflect what people generally eat at one time. For example, a pint of ice cream is now considered to contain three servings instead of four. When reading these labels, it is important to determine what constitutes a serving, as you might then eat more or less.

FAT

Fat functions in the body as a source of energy and also as a storage form of energy. It provides more calories per gram than carbohydrates or proteins: a gram of fat yields nine calories per gram compared with four for carbohydrate or protein. Fat protects the body's proteins by being metabolized (broken down) first to meet energy needs. It's necessary for the transport within the body of the essential vitamins A, D, E, and K, known as fat-soluble vitamins. Fat helps to maintain body temperature by providing insulation for the body.

In the past, it was assumed that a low-fat diet was the logical approach to weight loss. A low-fat diet would also help prevent heart disease since a high level of cholesterol, a naturally occurring fat in the body, is a major risk factor for coronary artery disease. It was also thought that the diet should be low in cholesterol, since doing so should lower cholesterol levels.

Low-fat diets have not been particularly effective, however. Their popularity may have contributed to widespread weight gain because, if your focus is mainly avoiding fat, it is easy to overconsume carbohydrates on a low-fat diet. The American Heart Association recommends that 25–35 percent of the calories in your diet come from fat.[1] **Some types of fat are much safer than others.**

To follow this, you need to understand just a dash of chemistry. Organic compounds, including those in food, have carbon atoms in their structure, and carbon atoms are connected with double bonds. Hydrogen atoms can be inserted between the carbon atoms either naturally or during the food manufacturing process, eliminating the double bond. If all of the carbons in a molecule are linked by hydrogen atoms rather than double bonds, the molecule is said to be "saturated" with hydrogen, hence the term "saturated fat." *Trans* fats have hydrogen atoms added by an industrial process, known as partial hydrogenation, and this results in the placement of hydrogen atoms on opposite sides of the double bond (*trans* configuration). In nature, most fats with hydrogen atoms between the carbon atoms have them on the same side (*cis* configuration), a more symmetrical arrangement. Figure 19.3 shows the *cis* and *trans* forms of a small molecule (not a fat).

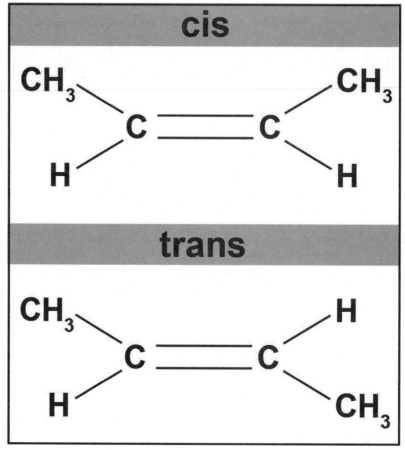

Figure 19.3. The *cis* and *trans* forms of 2-butene. C is carbon and H is hydrogen. Note that the *cis* form has both CH₃ groups on the same side of the double bond (the two parallel lines), whereas in the *trans* form they are on opposite sides.
Source: Shannon Simpson, *Cis-Trans Forms of 2-Butene,* July 2016. © Archaeopteryx Media LLC.

Another way of thinking about *cis* and *trans* is that since both of your ears point in the same direction, they are in the *cis* position. The barn owl, a nocturnal hunter, needs an exquisite sense of hearing and has one ear pointing up and one pointing down,[2] the *trans* position.

Trans fats are shown on both the previous and the new versions of the nutrition facts label (figure 19.2). Trans fats raise the unhealthy form of cholesterol (LDL cholesterol), lower the healthy form (HDL cholesterol), and increase the risk of heart disease and stroke.[3]

Table 19.1 shows that a healthy diet will contain fat but very little saturated fat and almost no trans fat. The American Heart Association has recom-

Table 19.1. Types of Fat

	Chemical Definition	Health Effects	Foods Containing This Type	Recommended Percentage of Calories within Diet
Monounsaturated	Contains one double bond between carbons	Reduces LDL (bad) cholesterol; source of vitamin E	Olive oil, canola oil, sesame oil, peanut oil	20–30% from mono- or polyunsaturated fats
Polyunsaturated*	Contains more than one double bond connecting carbons	Same as above	Soybean, corn, and sunflower oils; salmon, trout, herring	Same as above
Saturated	No double bonds between carbons	Raises cholesterol and promotes weight gain	Animal products, including red meat, butter, and cheese; palm, palm kernel, or coconut oils	5–10%
Trans**	Hydrogen atoms added to vegetable oils by industrial process	Raises LDL (bad) cholesterol and lowers HDL (good) cholesterol; increased risk of heart disease, stroke, and type 2 diabetes	Fried and baked foods. For example: doughnuts, frozen pizza, cakes, cookies, pie crusts, some stick margarine, many snack items	Less than 1%

*Includes omega-3 fatty acids, which are contained in fish and provide many health benefits.
Trans fats are listed in food ingredients as **partially hydrogenated oils.

mended that saturated fats be limited to 5–6 percent of calories consumed,[4] whereas the recently released *2015–2020 Dietary Guidelines for Americans*[5] (see box after the protein section) advise a limit of 10 percent. The generally accepted view is that limiting saturated fat is associated with a reduction in heart disease,[6] but some authorities argue that the evidence for a benefit in reducing saturated fat is weak.[7] **There is a great need for more and better quality studies on the health effects of diet.**

The new dietary guidelines also eliminated the limit on dietary cholesterol, but people are nevertheless advised to keep cholesterol to a minimum because many foods that are high in cholesterol are also high in saturated fat.

CARBOHYDRATES

Carbohydrates, commonly referred to as carbs, are an immediate energy source. Excess carbohydrates can be stored as fat. In much the same way as fats, carbohydrates are utilized preferentially to proteins. The basic unit of carbohydrates is a simple sugar (monosaccharide), and all complex carbs must be broken down to simple sugar to be absorbed. Carbs are classified by the number of sugar units. Carbs are part of the structure of DNA (the genetic material in the cells of the body) and other complex molecules. Carbohydrates are necessary for normal fat metabolism.

Carbohydrates occur naturally in many foods. Common examples of natural sugars are fructose in fruit, lactose in milk, and starch in potatoes. Carbohydrates may be refined (or processed), common examples being table sugar and high-fructose corn syrup. Carbs are stored as glycogen in humans and animals, mainly in the liver and in muscle, and as starch in plants. Almost all types of dietary fiber are carbohydrates.

While carbohydrates are necessary, overconsumption of them is a major factor in the high prevalence of weight gain and obesity in the United States today. The main culprit in the obesity epidemic is sugar that is added to foods in the manufacturing process to sweeten the taste, as opposed to sugars occurring naturally in foods. This *added sugar* comes with no vitamins, minerals, or other nutrients and provides no nutritional value other than adding more calories. Added sugar is found in sodas, fruit drinks, other sugary drinks, donuts, cookies, cakes, candy, sauces, dressings, ketchup, flavored yogurt, and dairy desserts.[8] **The new nutrition facts label (see figure 19.2) shows added sugar in both grams and % daily value. Added sugars are a subset of total sugars. The previous version of the nutrition facts label, which is being phased out, only shows total carbohydrates, whether natural or added. To determine if a food contains added sugar using the old label,**

look for the following in the ingredients list: agave nectar, any sugar, high-fructose corn syrup, honey, molasses, other syrup, and anything ending in –ose. A major change in the new dietary guidelines (see box after protein section) is the advice to restrict added sugars to less than 10 percent of the calories consumed.[9]

Sugars have four calories per gram. To calculate the number of carbohydrate calories in a serving, multiply the grams of carbohydrates in a serving by four.

FIBER

Dietary fiber is the non-digestible component of plant-derived foods.[10,11] Almost all fiber is carbohydrate and polysaccharide. Although fiber cannot be digested, some types can be fermented by the normal bacteria of the colon. For example, resistant starch is fermentable, whereas other types (e.g., cellulose) are not fermented and pass out in the stool unchanged. Fiber is found in fruits, vegetables, legumes, whole grains, nuts, and seeds. Fiber confers health benefits for the GI tract and may be helpful in treating or preventing diabetes and heart disease. Most Americans do not consume enough fiber; the recommended daily intake is 25 grams per day for women and 38 grams per day for men,[12] but the typical intake in adults in the United States is only 15 grams per day.[13]

Fiber has been subdivided in several ways:[14]

- Viscous and non-viscous
- Fermentable and non-fermentable

Table 19.2. Effects and Examples of Types of Fiber[15]

	Effects	Examples
Viscous	Forms a thick gel in water, slows emptying of stomach; reduces cholesterol levels; gas production	Pectins, beta-glucans, guar gum, mucilages (psyllium) Foods: legumes, wheat, rye, and oats
Nonviscous	Good laxative effect and less gas production	Cellulose, some hemicelluloses
Fermentable	Broken down to short-chain fatty acids, which can be absorbed and metabolized, and gas	Pectins, beta-glucans, guar gum, inulin Foods: oats, barley, legumes, some fruits, and vegetables
Non-fermentable	Good laxative effect and little gas production	Cellulose Foods: wheat bran (limited fermentation); nuts, seeds, skin of fruits, and vegetables

Fiber has also been characterized as soluble or insoluble, but the solubility of fiber has not been found to correlate with biochemical or functional features.[16] Fortunately, most fiber-containing foods contain more than one type, and increasing the overall amount of fiber in the diet is much more important than picking specific types. Fiber from food is generally more effective than fiber from supplements, although the latter, especially psyllium, can be beneficial. Beneficial health effects of increased fiber for which there is evidence include the following:

- Improved serum lipid levels, including LDL cholesterol
- Reduced risk of coronary heart disease
- Reduction in blood pressure and levels of inflammatory markers
- Improved blood glucose control in type 1 and 2 diabetes
- Reduced risk of developing type 2 diabetes
- Improvement in constipation, with softer stools, greater stool bulk, and shorter transit time (the time it takes for food to go through)

Gas production may increase with fiber-containing foods or supplements. Generous water intake is important for maximum benefit from fiber.[17]

Increasing intake of fiber, especially by food, may contribute to weight reduction, although the data are not conclusive. High-fiber foods often have fewer calories than their alternatives. Fiber can increase the feeling of fullness (satiety) after a meal, resulting in fewer calories being consumed. It may also decrease the absorption of nutrients from the small bowel.

Practical suggestions for increasing fiber intake:[18,19]

- Substitute or use whole grains in place of refined grains.
- For breakfast, eat oatmeal, whole-grain cereal, or bran cereal.
- For snacks, try low-fat popcorn, raw vegetables, fresh fruits, and nuts.
- Add legumes: beans, split peas, or lentils.
- Add cut-up vegetables to soups or sauces.
- Aim for five servings of fruits and vegetables per day.

Note: Make these changes slowly, and drink lots of water.

PROTEIN

It is recommended that 15–25 percent of your calories come from protein. Protein is found in animal and plant-derived foods. Animal protein may contain significant amounts of fat, including saturated fat and sodium. Excessive consumption of red meat, especially processed red meat, is associated with an increased risk of heart disease and cancer.[20,21] Protein from poultry, fish, or legumes is associated with less risk. Beans, lentils, or peas (legumes) are excellent protein sources.

THE 2015–2020 DIETARY GUIDELINES

On January 7, 2016, the U.S. Departments of Health and Human Services and Agriculture released the eighth edition of the *Dietary Guidelines for Americans*.[22] Guidelines on diet are released every five years as required by law, and they aim to keep the food supply safe and healthy. The dietary guidelines form the basis of federal programs such as the National School Lunch Program and the Special Supplemental Nutrition Program for Women, Infants, and Children (known as WIC).[23] Also, they are meant to encourage food manufacturers to make their products more healthy.[24]

Although much of the advice is unchanged from previous versions, the key changes include the following:[25,26]

- Calories from added sugars should be reduced so that they comprise 10 percent of calories per day.
- The limit on dietary cholesterol has been removed, but people are advised to keep cholesterol intake to a minimum because foods with cholesterol may contain saturated fat as well.
- Saturated fat should be less than 10 percent of calories per day.
- Sodium should be limited to 2,300 mg per day, as too much leads to elevated blood pressure. Spices, such as allspice, can be an alternative to salt.

The new guidelines have been criticized because they do not restrict red or processed meat,[27] although they do encourage protein from lean meats, seafood, poultry, eggs, legumes, nuts, seeds, and soy products.

PROBIOTICS, PREBIOTICS, AND THE MICROBIOME

These concepts may revolutionize our knowledge of digestive function and greatly enhance our ability to make positive changes.

Probiotics

Probiotics are living microorganisms (usually bacteria or yeast) that are intended to improve or maintain health. Probiotics can be taken in food or as a supplement. See chapter 9, "Irritable Bowel Syndrome," for precautions when taking probiotics as supplements. Yogurt is the most well-known probiotic-containing food, with kefir increasing in popularity. Probiotic foods are generally regarded as safe by the FDA and as such are not regulated or subject to much research.[28]

KEFIR

- A fermented milk product.
- "Kefir grain" refers to a soft mass of bacteria and yeast resembling cauliflower that can ferment milk.
- The bacterial and yeast composition of kefir is variable, but all contain lactobacillus bacteria that can digest lactose in milk. Kefir can usually be tolerated by people with lactose intolerance.
- The yeast in kefir produces carbon dioxide and ethanol, creating a beverage that is slightly sour, carbonated, and alcoholic (1–2 percent). Commercial preparations have the alcohol removed.
- Kefir is a good source of calcium and magnesium.
- Using kefir grains, kefir can be made at home from any type of milk, coconut milk (non-dairy), or even water.

Prebiotics

"Prebiotics" is a general term for components of food that humans cannot digest but that can be digested by our own bacteria in the intestinal tract, and that can provide beneficial changes in our bacterial population. Prebiotics are fermentable carbohydrates that can be oligosaccharides or polysaccharides, including fermentable fiber. Fermentable oligosaccharides are by definition FODMAPs and will not be tolerated by many with IBS (see chapter 9, "Irritable Bowel Syndrome").

The practical value of the prebiotic designation is dubious, since there are few data on which bacteria are stimulated by which prebiotics, what changes actually occur, and the benefits of such changes. Rather than looking for prebiotics, it is best to consume a wide variety of high-fiber foods.

PREBIOTICS, PROBIOTICS, AND SYNBIOTICS

- Prebiotics are carbohydrates that stimulate the growth or activity of existing bowel bacteria, leading to a health benefit.
- Probiotics are additional bowel bacteria that are added through food or supplements with the goal of achieving a health benefit.
- Synbiotics are a combination of prebiotics and probiotics. Prebiotics are said to be nutrition for the probiotics.

The Microbiome

The microbiome, or microbiota, refers to all of the microorganisms—bacteria, yeast, viruses, and parasites—that live on or in the human body. They can be located on or in the skin, nose, mouth, vagina, and the GI tract. The gut microbes reside mainly in the lower (distal) small intestine or in the colon. There are trillions of microbes in the human body, and they comprise ten times the number of cells that the human body contains.[29] Very little is known about the human microbiome, and most of the organisms in our bodies have not been cultured (grown in the laboratory) or otherwise identified, because the necessary conditions cannot be reproduced in the laboratory.[30]

As discussed earlier, the GI tract microbiome plays an important role in digestion via fermentation of carbohydrates that our own enzymes cannot metabolize. This may produce gas, which we generally regard as unpleasant, but there are also beneficial effects of fermentation. Fermentation causes the production of short-chain fatty acids that can be absorbed and metabolized, and one of these, butyrate, is the primary source of energy for the cells lining the colon.

Interest in the microbiome has increased as a result of recent experience with *Clostridium difficile* (*C. difficile,* or C-diff) infection (see also chapter 11, "*Clostridium difficile* Infection, or C-diff"). Normally, the microbiome keeps C-Diff, a minor component, in check. When the normal microbiome is reduced by antibiotic therapy, C-diff can overgrow in the colon and cause serious disease. The transfer of normal stool from a healthy donor to a patient with C-diff infection, a process known as fecal microbiota transplant, or stool transplant, has been enormously successful in treating patients who have not responded to other measures. Scientists are looking at the role of the microbiome in inflammatory bowel disease and other GI disorders. Some people with difficult-to-treat GI disorders have resorted to trying fecal microbiota transplants on their own, using stool from friends or family and protocols from the Internet, but the scientific support for this does not exist at this time and it cannot be recommended.

It is likely that study of the microbiome will lead to better treatments for many disorders, including those outside the GI tract. For example, transplantation of microbiota from a lean person to an obese person was associated with a temporary improvement in the ability of insulin to control blood sugar levels.[31]

In 2008, the National Institutes of Health initiated the Human Microbiome Project, an ambitious effort to study the human microbiome.[32,33] Great advances in our knowledge are anticipated.

THE HUMAN MICROBIOME PROJECT

The major goals of the project are:

- To determine the genetic sequences of 3,000 bacteria in human body sites, the largest group of which will be from the gut. These data will allow the study of microbial communities and provide a baseline for future research.
- Studies of the microbial communities at each body site to start to determine if there is a core group of organisms at each site.
- Studies of the relationship of changes in the human microbiome and disease.
- To develop new technology for data analysis.
- To assess the ethical, legal, and social aspects of microbiome research.

DIETS

Let's look at a few popular diets and then the best advice for healthy eating.

Gluten-Free Diets

A gluten-free diet is the only treatment for celiac disease (see chapter 15, "Disorders of the Stomach and Small Intestine, Including Celiac Disease") for details on the gluten-free diet) and strict, lifetime adherence is recommended. The diet eliminates wheat, barley, rye, and (at least initially) oats. A gluten-free diet has become widely popular among many in the general population who have adopted it to lose weight, improve athletic performance, feel better, or maintain a healthy lifestyle. It is estimated that 30 percent or more of Americans have tried a gluten-free diet.[34] The market for gluten-free foods is growing, and sales were estimated to reach $4 billion in 2015.[35]

Many people who do not have celiac disease have noted improvement in GI symptoms on a gluten-free diet. These individuals have been diagnosed as having *non-celiac gluten sensitivity*. It's tempting to speculate that many people with non-celiac gluten sensitivity may actually have IBS and are responding to the elimination of FODMAPs (see chapter 9, "Irritable Bowel Syndrome"). Other responders to a gluten-free diet may be as-yet-undiagnosed celiac patients. The diagnosis of celiac disease is made with blood antibody tests and biopsies of the small intestine done during an EGD (see chapter 13, "Evaluation of the Esophagus, Stomach, and Small Intestine"). When a person with celiac disease who does not know that he or she has it then starts a gluten-free diet before undergoing testing, the abnormal tests will improve and may become normal, and celiac disease may then be difficult to diagnose with certainty.

> If you are going gluten-free, get tested for celiac disease first. This is essential if you are trying the diet for symptom relief.

Is a gluten-free diet healthy for those without celiac disease? Not necessarily. In order to improve taste, some food manufacturers have added sugar or starch to gluten-free foods, especially processed ones, potentially adding to the calorie intake.[36] By their food choices, gluten-free enthusiasts may be unwittingly adding more calories, including unhealthy types. A gluten-free diet may be significantly lower in fiber, protein, vitamins, and minerals when many processed foods are used. Constipation may result from insufficient dietary fiber. Gluten-free adherents may need to compensate for the loss of whole grains by adding permitted whole grains such as quinoa and brown rice. A dietitian who specializes in teaching the gluten-free diet will provide guidance with correct choices and how to meet nutrient needs.

The Paleo Diet

The Paleo Diet seeks to reproduce the diet of our ancient ancestors, the cave men and women. It allows animal protein (meat and poultry), fish, eggs, fruits, vegetables, and some nuts. This diet allows much more meat than most others. The Paleo Diet does not permit grains, carbohydrates (except in fruit), potatoes, refined vegetable oils, or refined sugar. Processed foods are excluded, as are milk, dairy products, and legumes. Proponents of the Paleo Diet say that weight loss is likely because the diet is filling. There is no requirement to count calories or limit portions.

The Paleo Diet is low in carbohydrates, but it may be insufficient in fiber and high in fat, especially saturated fat. Eating red meat, especially processed red meat, may predispose one to heart disease and cancer, and red meat is unrestricted in the Paleo Diet. The exclusion of whole grains, which can lower cholesterol levels, may add to the increased heart disease risk. If carbohydrate intake is too low, the body will not be able to metabolize fat completely. There may be inadequate intake of calcium, magnesium, and vitamin D. Vitamin and mineral supplements may be needed.

Low-Carbohydrate (Atkins and Others)

Some of the concerns with the Paleo Diet apply to low carbohydrate diets: there may be too much fat (including saturated fat) and not enough fiber. Vitamin D may be deficient, and vitamin and mineral supplements may be needed. Low-carbohydrate diets are also difficult to maintain over a long period of time.

THE ESSENTIAL ELEMENTS OF HEALTHY EATING

- High-fiber diet using fruits, vegetables, salads, legumes, and whole grains
- Fish eaten twice a week
- Low-fat dairy products
- Limited red meat
- Limited added sugar (look in ingredients for any syrup, cane sugar, molasses, honey, high-fructose corn syrup, and anything ending in –ose)
- Limited saturated fat
- Little or no trans fat (look for partially hydrogenated oils in ingredients list)
- Proper balance of food groups
- **Regular exercise**

SOME NOTES ABOUT EXERCISE

- Start with regular, continuous walking at a steady, comfortable pace. Walking while at work or with the dog is less valuable because it is not sustained.
- Schedule your walking sessions five times per week, as you would an important appointment.
- You may go shopping to buy comfortable walking shoes.
- Walk up to fifteen to twenty minutes per session, and gradually increase the pace.
- After completing the above, discuss with your family physician the types of more intense exercise that would be appropriate for you. Consider cycling, swimming, jogging, running, water aerobics, and resistance training. A combination of these is ideal.
- Join your local gym or recreation center.
- If you can afford it and need more guidance, get a certified personal trainer.

GENERAL COMMENTS ABOUT WEIGHT REDUCTION

- Take steps to improve food choices; don't diet. Most people don't stick with diets.
- Avoiding added sugar is key. Healthy carbs from fruits and whole grains are best.
- Look carefully at your portion sizes. Consider using a smaller plate.
- Being overweight or obese is a chronic problem. A quick fix will not work. Develop a program that you can live with. The best results come from a sustained effort.
- Supermarket produce sections are excellent sources for finding fresh fruits and vegetables.
- Many diets will result in a noticeable loss of weight in the early stages. As time goes on, the body adapts to the dietary change, and further weight loss may be slower. The body may have "reset its thermostat" during the period that the weight was higher and may function as if the higher weight is the norm. This will take more time to improve.
- Exercise is an essential component of a weight loss program.
- For severe obesity, bariatric surgery can be effective. Diabetes may disappear and blood pressure can become normal. Discuss this with your family physician and gastroenterologist. Research it carefully, as there are risks.
- Set realistic goals for your body image. Move away from the stereotypes promoted by Hollywood, the media, and the fashion industry.

HEALTHY EATING SUMMARY: TEN POINTS TO SUCCESS

1. Define your goals: is it weight loss to improve symptoms, to maintain health, or other reasons? Research ways to accomplish your goal.
2. Keep a food and symptom diary.
3. Start reading ingredient labels. Learn the meaning of the terms used.
4. Decrease consumption of foods with added sugars.
5. Avoid saturated and trans fat.
6. Exercise regularly. Even a small increase in physical activity is good for you.
7. Get evaluated for celiac disease before eliminating gluten from your diet.
8. Cut back on processed foods. Go natural. Make better choices when shopping or eating out.
9. Keep a good balance of fat (25–35 percent), carbohydrates (40–55 percent), and protein (15–25 percent).
10. Consult with a licensed dietitian for best results.

WHAT ABOUT SUPPLEMENTS?

People often assume that herbal and dietary supplements are safe and that they provide health benefits. In reality, supplements can cause significant harm. In a recent study, all liver injuries related to drugs (conventional medications or supplements) from 2004 to 2013 were examined.[37] Herbal products were included in the supplement group. The key findings were as follows:

- One hundred thirty of 839 instances of drug-related injury over this ten-year period seen at eight U.S. referral centers were caused by supplements (15.5 percent). The other 709 patients had liver injury from medications.
- The percentage of episodes related to supplements increased from 7 to 20 percent from 2004 to 2013.
- Of the 130 injuries related to supplements, 45 occurred in bodybuilders, but there were no deaths or need for liver transplantation in this group.
- Among the non-bodybuilders with supplement-related liver injury, middle-aged women predominated. Deaths or need for liver transplantation were more frequent (13 percent) in non-bodybuilders using supplements than in those with liver injury from medications (3 percent).

> Consult a physician before taking dietary or herbal supplements.

Some supplements used by non-bodybuilders that have caused serious or fatal liver injury[38] include:

- Black cohosh
- Chaparral
- Chaso
- Germander
- He Shou Wu
- Hydroxycut
- Kava kava
- Licorice
- Noni juice
- Onshido
- Pennyroyal

TAKE-HOME MESSAGES

- See the healthy eating summary above.
- See previous sections for tips on healthy eating, exercise, and weight reduction.
- Do not assume that dietary supplements and herbal products are harmless. Research any that you take, and discuss them with your physician.

20

How to Get the Most out of Your Visit to the Doctor

Patients' complaints about physicians are well known and include long waiting times, a physician who does not listen, and unprofessional conduct. Among the medical stories that went viral in 2015 was an incident in which an anesthesiologist made disparaging remarks about a patient while he was sedated for colonoscopy,[1] obviously an unacceptable behavior. There is little written, however, on what patients can do to make their visits to the doctor more productive. Here are some tips on how to do that:

1. Come prepared for your visit. Your doctor has set aside time for you, so take a few minutes to do some pre-appointment homework.
2. Prepare a document of your medical history, including past illnesses, operations, allergies, medications, and family history. Include your pharmacy name and number. It is preferable to keep this on your computer for easy updating. Bring an updated document to each visit.
3. Think about your most important complaint and write it down. Your doctor can help you most if you can be concise. Think about ways to characterize your complaint. Where is it located? When did it start? How long does it last? How severe is it? Try to keep what you say relevant to your reason for coming in.
4. If you have pain, your doctor will also want to know the type of pain: burning, sharp, dull, aching, pressure-like, stabbing, etc. Think about the various types of pain and write down the word(s) that best describe yours. Sometimes this can be difficult, but describing the quality of pain can be very helpful. When your doctor asks you about the type of pain, try not to say, "It hurts," or "It's really bad."

5. Consider whether there are any other symptoms that are associated with the main complaint, and write them down. For example, "Whenever I get a squeezing pain just below the ribs on the right side, I also have nausea."

6. You may have other symptoms which do not appear related to the main complaint. Write a list of your complaints in the order of importance, and discuss them in this order.

7. Look over your notes and think about what you want to say. It is okay to bring your notes with you to the office and have them in front of you when you are speaking to the doctor.

8. After you have given over your main complaints, your doctor may ask additional questions about them. Since he or she may have a particular diagnosis in mind when asking the question, it is important that you answer the question as it was asked. As much as your doctor might want to hear more details, your background information is best kept brief.

9. Remember that being prepared for an appointment helps to keep your doctor on schedule so you and other patients can be seen in a timely way.

10. When scheduling a visit, keep the following two hours after the visit open. There are legitimate reasons why doctors "run late." Doctors do get emergencies. Sometimes other patients come in on the wrong day. An earlier patient may have been late, backing up everyone else. Often, other patients need extra time; sometimes, you may need extra time. Electronic medical records take more time. There are some doctors who intentionally overbook, but hopefully you can figure this out. When scheduling a procedure, make sure that your driver has similar flexibility.

11. If you have been waiting a long time, it is okay to ask someone in the office how much longer it will be. After a very long wait, you may be tempted to walk out, but definitely check with someone before doing so.

12. Know your medications, including over-the-counter medications. Know their names and the ailments for which they are used. Learn to pronounce their names. Don't say, "I take a little white pill." Or, a blue pill, a teal pill, a chartreuse pill, etc. Alternatively, keep a list of all of your medications in your wallet, which will be readily available to hand over to your doctor or office staff so they can copy it and enter it into your medical record.

13. Know your allergies, including the name of the drug and what happened when you took it. Avoid being in the position of having to say, "I'm allergic to antibiotics."

14. Be honest about your alcohol and drug use. Your doctor cannot help you if he or she does not have accurate information. I'll let you in on a trade secret: in medical school, students are taught to double the quantity of alcohol that the patient admits to drinking each day.

15. Be aware that gastroenterologists will not with rare exceptions prescribe medications for pain. Decisions on analgesics (pain medications), especially opioids, which are habit forming, are best deferred to the primary care physician in order to prevent patients from obtaining prescriptions from several doctors. Hydrocodone and oxycodone are examples of opioids. Another type of analgesic that gastroenterologists will usually not prescribe is the non-steroidal, anti-inflammatory drugs (ibuprofen, naproxen, diclofenac, and others) because of their ability to cause ulcers or erosions in the stomach or elsewhere in the GI tract.

16. Provide a list, not only of prescription drugs, but also herbal medications, supplements, vitamins, and alternative medications.

17. When your doctor prescribes a new medication, ask if it is compatible with those that you are already taking.

18. You can and should ask questions. You may bring a list of these.

19. You do not have to accept every recommendation. Ask about alternatives. Ask about radiation exposure, especially if you have had several CT scans and other imaging procedures involving radiation. If the advice you receive does not sound right, consider another opinion. A good doctor is not threatened by your interest in a second opinion; in fact, he or she may welcome it.

BONUS TIP FOR THE HOSPITAL

Patients who are hospitalized, and especially those receiving antibiotics in the hospital, may acquire an infection with *Clostridium difficile* (see also chapter 11, "*Clostridium difficile* Infection, or C-diff"). This bacteria, commonly referred to as C-diff, causes diarrhea, which can be severe. C. diff can be difficult to eradicate, in part because it forms spores which may be spread by hands or stethoscopes. The common alcohol-based hand rubs seen everywhere in hospitals do not kill the C. diff spores. Hand washing with soap and water for at least fifteen seconds is more effective and is recommended. If you are hospitalized, politely ask all health care personnel to wash their hands in this way and to clean their stethoscopes. If C. diff is suspected, make sure that everyone entering your room complies with infection control precautions (gowns and gloves) and that surfaces are periodically cleaned with bleach or a comparable solution.

Acknowledgments

I am extremely grateful to the many wonderful people who provided encouragement, support, and skill during the writing of this book. In the beginning, when I knew little about writing or publishing outside of medical journals, and had no idea where to start, Amanda Avutu, Molly Campbell, Judy Gruen, Debbie Price, and Elizabeth Sammons pointed me in the right direction. Several people read earlier versions of this book, which had a different focus (medical humor) but which set the stage for this work. I am indebted to Kate Carlisle; Doris Fickler RN; Kim Johnson; Martha Moody MD; Steve Rudich MD, PhD; Joan Servis; and Jeffrey Stoller.

Many kind individuals reviewed chapters of this book and provided literary or medical expertise, and I thank you all: Robyn Karlstadt MD; Robert Schaefer MD; Richard Houston MD; Deborah Stokes; Dinish Hassan PhD; Jayson Barnett MD; Monica Cengia RD; Evan Fisher MD; Jigna Thakore MD; Anjali Morey MD, PhD; Stephen Harris; Marie K. Hammond; Marios Pouagare MD, PhD; Narayan Peddanna MD; Urmee Siraj MD; Tristan Handler MD; Salma Akram MD; Anna S. Lok MD; Anne Marie Romer RN; Shannon Simpson; Juliet Glaser; Joan Servis; and Leora Novick.

Special thanks to Ellyn Miller and Shannon Simpson for artwork, Abigail Auxter of AmSurg Corp. and Brenda Reagan RN for help with the book proposal, Margaret Chappell of the Kettering Medical Center Library for keeping me well supplied with journal articles, Abida Mukhdomi MD for the story about the field hospital in India, and intellectual property attorney Stephen E. Gillen for answering numerous questions. I also thank the many medical personnel and patients who provided humorous anecdotes for the original incarnation of this book.

I could not have completed this work without the help of Melissa Schirmer of Mosaic Editing. Melissa's editing and formatting skills have made my work presentable and more readable.

Tremendous thanks to my agent, Veronica Park (Twitter handle Veroni-Kaboom—that says it all), whose boundless enthusiasm kept everything moving. I have great appreciation for Suzanne Stazak-Silva, executive editor at Rowman & Littlefield, whose sage advice kept this book focused on the important messages. Kathryn Knigge and Elaine McGarraugh, and many others at Rowman whose names I do not know, provided essential expertise.

My children, Batya and Orren Azani, and Elana, Aviva, and Leora Novick, provided on-target comments and needed encouragement at every stage of the writing process.

To my wife, Jane, for unfailingly accurate advice, and support in every way, above and beyond.

Notes

INTRODUCTION

1. American Cancer Society, "Cancer Facts 2016."
2. National Institutes of Health, "Cancer Costs."
3. National Institute of Diabetes and Digestive and Kidney Diseases, "Irritable Bowel Syndrome."
4. Centers for Disease Control and Prevention, "Epidemiology of the IBD."
5. Pemberton, "Colonic Diverticulosis."
6. American College of Gastroenterology, "Acid Reflux."
7. Bischoff, "Gut Health?"
8. Rinella and Charlton, "Globalization of Fatty Liver Disease," 19.
9. Younossi et al., "Global Epidemiology of Fatty Liver Disease," 73.
10. Anonymous, "Gut Health."
11. Brisebois, "Steal This!"
12. Kresser, "9 Steps to Perfect Health—#5: Heal Your Gut."
13. NIH Human Microbiome Project, "Microbiome Analyses."
14. Vindigni et al., "The Intestinal Microbiome, Barrier Function, and Immune System in Inflammatory Bowel Disease."
15. Quigley, "Leaky Gut: Concept or Clinical Entity," 74.

CHAPTER 1. PREPARING FOR COLONOSCOPY

1. Sweetser and Baron, "Optimizing Bowel Cleansing for Colonoscopy," 522.

CHAPTER 2. SEDATION AND ANESTHESIA

1. Associated Press, "Jackson's Death Officially Ruled a Homicide."
2. Gottlieb, "Michael Jackson Had Several Drugs."
3. McCartney, "Michael Jackson Death Certificate."
4. Medina, "Doctor Is Guilty in Michael Jackson's Death."
5. Ibid.
6. Gottlieb, "Michael Jackson Had Several Drugs."
7. Avila and Ng, "Michael Jackson's Doctor Guilty."

CHAPTER 5. PUTTING COLONOSCOPY IN PERSPECTIVE: THE EVIDENCE, QUALITY ISSUES, AND SURVEILLANCE INTERVALS

1. Swift, "Sessile Serrated Adenomas."
2. Strum, "Colorectal Adenomas," 1065.
3. American Cancer Society, "Cancer Facts 2016."
4. Ibid.
5. Siegel et al., "Colorectal Cancer Statistics, 2014" 104.
6. Winawer et al., "Prevention of Colorectal Cancer," 1977.
7. Zauber et al., "Colonoscopic Polypectomy," 687.
8. Siegel et al., "Colorectal Cancer Statistics."
9. Yang et al., "Colorectal Cancers Prevented," 2893.
10. Welch and Robertson, "Colorectal Cancer on the Decline," 1607.
11. Amri et al., "Impact of Screening Colonoscopy," 747.
12. Kahi et al., "Screening and Surveillance," 335.
13. Ibid.
14. Corley et al., "Adenoma Detection Rate," 1298.
15. Agrawal et al., "Colorectal Cancer in African Americans," 515.
16. Multi-Society Task Force, "Guidelines on Lynch Syndrome," 197.
17. Rex et al., "American College of Gastroenterology Guidelines," 739.
18. Qaseem et al., "Screening for Colorectal Cancer," 378.
19. Lieberman et al., "Guidelines for Colonoscopy," 844.
20. Strum, "Colorectal Adenomas."
21. Lieberman et al., "Guidelines for Colonoscopy."
22. van Hees et al., "Screening in Elderly Persons," 750.

CHAPTER 6. COLONOSCOPY: RISKS, ALTERNATIVES, AND BARRIERS

1. ASGE Standards of Practice Committee, "Complications of Colonoscopy," 745.

CHAPTER 7. OVERVIEW OF COLON CANCER

1. National Cancer Institute, "What Is Cancer?"
2. Ibid.
3. National Cancer Institute, "Targeted Therapy."
4. National Cancer Institute, "Targeted Cancer Therapy."
5. Goldstein and Mitchell, "Carcinoembryonic Antigen," 338.
6. Cleveland Clinic, "Overview of Colorectal Cancer."
7. Siegel et al., "Colorectal Cancer Statistics," 104.
8. Kahi et al., "Colonoscopy after Cancer Resection," 489.

CHAPTER 8. DIVERTICULOSIS AND DIVERTICULITIS

1. Markham and Li, "Diverticulitis of the Right Colon," 547.
2. Morris et al., "Sigmoid Diverticulitis," 287.
3. Strate et al., "Nut, Corn, and Popcorn Consumption," 907.
4. Morris et al., "Sigmoid Diverticulitis."
5. Shahedi et al., "Long-Term Risk of Acute Diverticulitis," 1609.
6. Morris et al., "Sigmoid Diverticulitis."
7. Ibid.
8. Kvasnovsky et al., "Increased Diverticular Complications," 189.

CHAPTER 9. IRRITABLE BOWEL SYNDROME

1. Ford et al., "Management of Irritable Bowel Syndrome," S2.
2. Ibid.
3. McKenzie et al., "British Dietetic Association Guidelines for Dietary Management," 260.
4. Shepherd and Gibson, *The Complete Low-FODMAP Diet*, 24.
5. Ong et al., "Pattern of Gas Production," 1366.
6. Halmos et al., "Diet Low in FODMAPS," 67.
7. Gibson and Shepherd, "Evidence-Based Dietary Management," 252.
8. Allergan.com, "Full Prescribing Information for Viberzi."

CHAPTER 10. CROHN'S DISEASE AND ULCERATIVE COLITIS (INFLAMMATORY BOWEL DISEASE)

1. Feagan et al., "Vedolizumab for Ulcerative Colitis," 699.
2. Sandborn et al., "Vedolizumab for Crohn's Disease," 711.

3. Cominelli, "Inhibition of Leukocyte Trafficking," 775.
4. Lobatón et al., "Anti-adhesion Therapies," 581.
5. Ibid., 582.
6. Picarella et al., "Monoclonal Antibodies Specific for β_7 Integrin," 2099.
7. www.goodrx.com.
8. FDA, "FDA Approves Inflectra."
9. Nielsen and Ainsworth, "Tumor Necrosis Factor Inhibitors," 754.
10. Elsagher, *I'd Like to Buy a Bowel, Please.*
11. Elsagher, *It's in the Bag and Under the Covers.*
12. Rutter and Riddell, "Colorectol Dysplasia," 359.
13. Laine et al. "Management of Dysplasia," 651.
14. ASGE Standards of Practice Committee, "The Role of Endoscopy," 1101.
15. Ibid.

CHAPTER 11. *CLOSTRIDIUM DIFFICILE* INFECTION, OR C-DIFF

1. Lessa et al., "Burden of *Clostridium difficile*," 825.
2. Ibid.
3. Bagdasarian et al., "Diagnosis and Treatment of *Clostridium difficile*," 401.
4. Ibid., 399.
5. Ibid.
6. Ibid.
7. C Diff Foundation, "*C. difficile* Care at Home."
8. Vermont Department of Health, "Living with C. Diff."
9. Leffler and Lamont, "*Clostridium difficile* Infection," 1539.
10. www.goodrx.com.
11. Bagdasarian et al., "Diagnosis and Treatment of *Clostridium difficile*," 405.
12. www.goodrx.com.
13. Bagdasarian et al., "Diagnosis and Treatment of *Clostridium difficile*," 405
14. van Nood et al., "Duodenal Infusion of Donor Feces," 407.
15. Lee et al., "Frozen vs Fresh Fecal Microbiota Transplantation," 142.

CHAPTER 13. EVALUATION OF THE ESOPHAGUS, STOMACH, AND SMALL INTESTINE

1. Kovaleva et al., "Transmission of Infection," 231.
2. Meyer, "Endoscope Disinfection."
3. Marcus, "Joan Rivers' Cause of Death."
4. Duke, "Joan Rivers Died from 'Therapeutic Complications.'"
5. Hartocollis, "Joan Rivers Died from Complication."
6. Rizzo, "What Really Happened to Joan Rivers."
7. Italiano and Marsh, "Unplanned Biopsy Led to Joan Rivers' Death?"

8. Singer, "Did Joan Rivers Die of VIP Syndrome?"

9. Epstein et al., "Exposure to Duodenoscopes," 1447

10. Rutala and Weber, "Gastrointestinal Endoscopes," 1405.

11. Kim et al., "Risk Factors Associated with Transmission," 1121.

12. Ibid.

CHAPTER 14. HEARTBURN AND REFLUX

1. American College of Gastroenterology, "Acid Reflux."

2. Yang et al., "Risk of Hip Fracture," 2947.

3. Schoenfeld and Grady, "Adverse Effects Associated with Proton Pump Inhibitors," 172.

4. Lazarus et al., "Risk of Chronic Kidney Disease," 238.

5. Antoniou et al., "Risk of Acute Kidney Injury," E166.

6. Schoenfeld and Grady, "Adverse Effects Associated with Proton Pump Inhibitors."

7. Gomm et al., "Association of Proton Pump Inhibitors with Risk of Dementia," 410.

8. Haenisch et al., "Risk of Dementia in Elderly Patients," 419.

9. Kuller, "Do Proton Pump Inhibitors Increase the Risk?" 379.

10. Gomm et al., "Association of Proton Pump Inhibitors with Risk of Dementia,"

11. Katz, "Failing the Acid Test," 747.

12. Furuta and Katzka, "Eosinophilic Esophagitis," 1640.

13. Desai et al., "Esophageal Food Impaction," 795.

14. Spechler and Souza, "Barrett's Esophagus," 836.

15. Ibid.

16. Rubenstein et al., "Prediction of Barrett's Esophagus," 353.

17. American Cancer Society, "Cancer Facts and Figures 2016."

18. Pohl et al., "Esophageal Adenocarcinoma Incidence," 1468.

19. Engel et al., "Population Attributable Risks," 1404.

20. American Cancer Society, "How Is Cancer of the Esophagus Staged?"

CHAPTER 15. DISORDERS OF THE STOMACH AND SMALL INTESTINE, INCLUDING CELIAC DISEASE

1. Hasler, "Gastric Emptying," 208.

2. Richter et al., "*Helicobacter pylori* and Gastroesophageal Reflux Disease," 1800.

3. Oxemtenko and Murray, "Celiac Disease," 1396.

4. Kelly and Dennis, "Patient Information."

5. Dunavan, "Reading Gluten-Free Labels."

6. Mayo Clinic Staff, "Gluten-Free Diet."

7. Thalheimer, "Gluten-Free Whole Grains."

8. Getz, "Gluten-Free Fast Food."
9. Gluten-Free Living, "Eating at Restaurants."
10. Moran, "Eating Gluten-Free at Restaurants."
11. Schaeffer, "Gluten-Free Appetizers."

CHAPTER 16. GALLBLADDER AND PANCREAS

1. Cotton et al., "Gallbladder and Sphincter of Oddi Disorders," 1420.
2. Cafasso and Smith, "Functional Disorders of the Biliary Tract," 237.
3. Banks et al., "Classification of Acute Pancreatitis," 103.
4. Working Group IAP/APA, "Management of Acute Pancreatitis," e5.
5. Canto et al., "Cancer of the Pancreas Screening (CAPS) Consortium," 339.

CHAPTER 17. HEPATITIS C

1. Reau, "HCV Testing," 31.
2. Centers for Disease Control and Prevention, "Hepatitis C."
3. Denniston et al., "Chronic Hepatitis C," 293.
4. AASLD-IDSA, "HCV Testing and Linkage to Care."
5. Cicero et al., "The Changing Face of Heroin Use," 821.
6. Novick and Novick, "Fight Ohio's Heroin Epidemic," 17.
7. Novick and Kreek, "Treatment of Hepatitis C," 905.
8. Gabrielli et al., "Spread of Hepatitis C virus among Sexual Partners," 17.
9. Farci and Purcell, "Genotypes and Quasispecies," 103.
10. Smith et al., "Expanded Classification of Hepatitis C Virus," 318.
11. Manos et al., "Distribution of Hepatitis C Virus Genotypes," 1744.
12. McCombs et al., "The Risk of Long-Term Morbidity and Mortality," 204.
13. Ferrarese et al., "Liver Transplantation for Viral Hepatitis," 1570.
14. Bedossa et al., "Activity in Chronic Hepatitis C," 289.
15. Poynard et al., "Liver Fibrosis Progression," 730.
16. El-Serag, "Hepatocellular Carcinoma," 1118.
17. Afdhal et al., "Ledipasvir and Sofosbuvir," 1889.
18. AASLD-IDSA, "Recommendations for Testing."
19. AASLD-IDSA, "When and in Whom to Initiate HCV Therapy."
20. www.goodrx.com
21. Barua et al., "Restrictions for Medicaid Reimbursement of Sofosbuvir," 215.
22. Canary et al., "Limited Access to New Hepatitis C Virus Treatment," 226.
23. Ibid.
24. Center for Medicaid and CHIP Services, "Assuring Medicaid Beneficiaries Access."
25. United States Senate Committee on Finance, "Revenue-Driven Pricing."
26. Leidner et al., "Cost-Effectiveness of Hepatitis C Treatment," 1860.
27. Lowes, "First Drug for All Major Forms of HCV."

28. AASLD-IDSA. "Monitoring Patients."
29. Substance Abuse and Mental Health Services Administration, "Opioid Use Disorder."
30. Jones et al., "Opioid Agonist Medication-Assisted Treatment," e55.

CHAPTER 18. CIRRHOSIS AND THE SPECTRUM OF LIVER DISEASE

1. Xu et al., "Deaths," 8.
2. Xu et al., ibid.
3. Poynard et al., "Impact of Pegylated Interferon," 1303.
4. Novick et al., "Hepatic Cirrhosis in Young Adults," 8.
5. Hutchinson et al., "Influence of Alcohol," 1150.
6. Novick, "Corticosteroids as Therapeutic Agents," 30.
7. Rinella and Charlton, "Globalization of Fatty Liver Disease," 19.
8. Younossi et al., "Global Epidemiology of Fatty Liver Disease," 73.
9. Brooks, "FDA Clears Obeticholic Acid."
10. Corpechot, "Beyond Ursodeoxycholic Acid," 15.
11. Kamath et al., "Primary Biliary Cirrhosis," 1066.
12. Hayward et al., "Paracetamol (Acetaminophen)," 213.
13. Chopra, "Patient Information: Cirrhosis."
14. Hayward et al., "Paracetamol (Acetaminophen)."
15. Leung and Wong, "Medical Management of Ascites," 1269.
16. Wong, "Management of Ascites," 11.
17. Leung and Wong, "Medical Management of Ascites."
18. Wong, "Management of Ascites."
19. Angeli and Gines, "Hepatorenal Syndrome," 1135.
20. Ferenci et al., "Hepatic Encephalopathy," 716.
21. Patidar and Bajaj, "Covert and Overt Hepatic Encephalopathy," 2048.
22. Vierling, "Legal Responsibilities of Physicians," 577.
23. Lauridsen et al., "Driving Simulator Performance," 747.
24. Vierling, ibid.
25. Neff et al., "Durability of Rifaximin Response," 168.
26. Patel et al., "Hepatic Encephalopathy," 79.
27. Kachaamy and Bajaj, "Diet and Cognition," 174.
28. Ibid.
29. Kawaguchi et al., "Branched-Chain Amino Acids," 1063.
30. Shah et al., "Living Donor Liver Transplantation," 339.
31. United Network for Organ Sharing, "Living Donation."

CHAPTER 19. HEALTHY EATING

1. American Heart Association, "Know Your Fats."
2. Barn Owl Conservation Network, "Barn Owl's Sense of Hearing."

3. American Heart Association, "Trans Fats."

4. American Heart Association, "Saturated Fats."

5. U.S. Department of Health and Human Services and U.S. Department of Agriculture, *2015–2020 Dietary Guidelines*.

6. DeSalvo et al. "Dietary Guidelines for Americans," 457.

7. Nissen, "U.S. Dietary Guidelines," 558.

8. American Heart Association, "Added Sugars."

9. U.S. Department of Health and Human Services and U.S. Department of Agriculture, *2015–2020 Dietary Guidelines*.

10. Eswaran et al., "Fiber and Functional Gastrointestinal Disorders," 718.

11. Slavin, Position of the Diabetic Association, 1716.

12. Mayo Clinic, "Dietary Fiber."

13. Slavin, Position of the Diabetic Association.

14. Eswaran et al., "Fiber and Functional Gastrointestinal Disorders."

15. Slavin, Position of the Diabetic Association.

16. Higdon and Drake, "Fiber."

17. Novick, "Conquer Constipation."

18. Mayo Clinic, "Dietary Fiber."

19. Higdon and Drake, "Fiber."

20. International Agency for Research on Cancer, "Red Meat and Processed Meat."

21. Bouvard et al., "Carcinogenicity of Red and Processed Meat," 1599.

22. U.S. Department of Health and Human Services and U.S. Department of Agriculture, *2015–2020 Dietary Guidelines*.

23. Szabo, "Why New Dietary Guidelines Matter."

24. Hamburg, "Updates to the Nutrition Facts Label."

25. DeSalvo et al., "Dietary Guidelines for Americans."

26. Christenson. "New U.S. Dietary Guidelines Limit Sugar, Rethink Cholesterol."

27. Fox, "Who's Mad about the New Dietary Guidelines?"

28. Floch, "Probiotics and Prebiotics."

29. Yeager, "Mapping the Gut Microbiome."

30. NIH Human Microbiome Project, "Microbiome Analysis."

31. Vrieze et al., "Transfer of Intestinal Microbiota," 913.

32. Methé et al., "A Framework for Human Microbiome Research," 215.

33. NIH Human Microbiome Project, "Overview."

34. Getz, "Gluten-Free Fast Food."

35. Balistreri, "Should We All Go Gluten-Free?"

36. Voorhees and Durgin, "Gluten-Free."

37. Navarro et al., "Liver Injury from Herbals and Dietary Supplements," 1399.

38. Navarro and Lucena, "Hepatotoxicity Induced by Supplements," 172.

CHAPTER 20. HOW TO GET THE MOST
OUT OF YOUR VISIT TO THE DOCTOR

1. Jackman, "Anesthesiologist Trashes Sedated Patient."

Glossary

Within the definitions, terms in bold are defined elsewhere in the glossary.

abscess—A collection of pus in a cavity. A drainage procedure and antibiotics are usually needed.

acid reflux—See **GE reflux.**

acute—A symptom or condition that is intense, severe, or of short duration, in contrast to **chronic.**

adenocarcinoma—A malignant growth, or cancer, that arises from an **adenoma** or from **gland**ular tissue. Can occur in the **esophagus**, stomach, small intestine, **colon**, pancreas, and other sites.

adenoma—1. In the colon, a **benign polyp** with a small but definite risk of progression to cancer. **Villous adenomas** (see second definition) have increased risk. Adenomas in the **colon** grow out from the inner lining into the **lumen**. They may be flat or on a stalk. 2. **Benign** tumors (growths) elsewhere in the body. Adenomas are derived from glandular tissue. They grow much more slowly than cancer cells and do not spread through the blood or to adjacent tissues as cancers do.

adenoma detection rate—The proportion of patients undergoing screening colonoscopy in whom one or more **adenomas** are detected. The **adenoma** detection rate is used to assess physicians' performance of screening colonoscopy, to see how thorough the procedures are.

adenomatous polyp—A **polyp** that is an **adenoma.**

adjuvant chemotherapy—Medications prescribed after cancer surgery that is done with the intention to cure.

albumin—A protein that can dissolve in water and circulate in the blood. It is also found in egg whites. It is administered in conjunction with large-volume **paracentesis** for ascites and as a treatment for hepatorenal syndrome.

amino acid—An organic acid (found in living tissue) containing the amino group (NH_2). Amino acids are the major components of proteins. An *essential* amino acid cannot be made in the body, is necessary for the body's health, and must be obtained in the diet.

ammonia—A compound of hydrogen and nitrogen (NH_3) that is produced by GI tract bacteria. It can accumulate in liver disease, mainly **cirrhosis**, and contribute to **hepatic encephalopathy**.

Ampulla of Vater—The opening whereby the common bile duct and the pancreatic duct form a common channel and discharge their contents into the **duodenum**.

anal fissure—A tear or linear **ulcer** in the mucous membrane of the anus, which can be quite painful.

anesthesia—The loss of ability to feel pain along with the induction of a sleep-like state caused by administration of drugs by a trained health care professional. The patient usually has no memory of the events that occur during anesthesia.

anoscope—A small clear plastic **scope**, about two inches long, designed to visualize the anal canal.

antibody—A protein produced by certain white blood cells for the purpose of neutralizing a foreign substance, including bacteria and viruses.

anticoagulant—A medication that reduces the ability of blood to clot.

ascites—Fluid that accumulates in the abdominal cavity, sometimes in such large quantities that the patient has obvious visible abdominal distention. It is most commonly caused by **cirrhosis** of the liver but can also be a result of heart failure or kidney disease. It can accumulate to massive amounts and can be treated with drugs or removed by procedures.

aspiration—The inhalation of stomach contents that have traveled up the **esophagus** and into the throat; if they reach the lungs, aspiration pneumonia can result.

asterixis—a flapping tremor of the hands seen when the wrist is extended (as if you are motioning someone to stop). It is seen in hepatic encephalopathy, in all but the early stages.

autoantibody—An antibody directed against an organ or tissue of the patient's own body. They are seen in **autoimmune diseases** such as **autoimmune hepatitis**.

autoimmune disease—A disease in which the patient's own immune system attacks his or her own organs or body tissues. More than one organ may be affected.

autoimmune hepatitis—Liver inflammation caused by the patient's immune system reacting against the liver. This disorder can usually be effectively treated with medications but can lead to liver **cirrhosis**.

average risk—The risk for a disease in people with no known risk factors. For example, people with no family history of **colon** cancer or **adenomatous polyps** and no personal history of colon adenomas are considered to be average risk for **colon** cancer.

barium enema—X-rays of the **colon** after barium, an opaque contrast agent, has been instilled into the rectum in sufficient quantity to fill the colon. The patient must turn in various ways to obtain all of the images. Patients may complain about being on a hard table in awkward positions, bloating or discomfort during the exam, or trouble holding the barium in.

Barrett's esophagus—A condition in which there are changes in the cells of the **distal** (lower) esophagus so that they resemble those of the small intestine. These cells can develop **dysplasia** and cancer in some patients.

benign—Not malignant; not cancerous; usually associated with a good outcome.

benzodiazepines—A group of chemically related drugs which may be used for treatment of anxiety or insomnia; they are sedatives or minor tranquilizers. They may also be used to treat seizures, muscle spasms, or alcohol withdrawal. They are potentially habit forming, or addictive.

bezoar—A concretion of foreign material in the GI tract, especially the stomach. Bezoars most commonly consist of food or hair.

bile salts—A group of substances that originate in the liver, are stored in and secreted from the gallbladder, and digest fat in the GI tract. Bile salts are closely related to conjugated bile acids.

biliary colic—A dull, steady pain in the mid or right upper abdomen that is typical of gallbladder disease. It may also be felt in the right shoulder or back. It is not colic, which is a pain that waxes and wanes.

biologic drug—A drug that is manufactured in a biological system such as a bacteria or cell culture, rather than by a chemical process. Many biologic drugs are large, complex molecules that cannot be fully characterized in the laboratory. Because of this, a competing company may not be able to manufacture an identical molecule. **Generic** drugs, which must be exactly identical to the original, have not been approved for biologics in the United States. The Affordable Care Act contains a shortened approval pathway for **biosimilar** drugs, which are similar but not identical to the biologic drugs. The biologic drugs used in **Crohn's disease** and **ulcerative colitis** are **monoclonal antibodies** which block a receptor in the cell that is important in inflammation.

biopsy—A tissue sample, removed to diagnose a disease. Usually the tissue is stained with various dyes or chemicals to allow the features of the tissue to be clear to the physician examining it under a microscope. A biopsy does NOT mean cancer; it may be performed to rule out cancer. Cancer is one of the many findings that can be seen under the microscope.

biosimilar—A **biologic drug** that has the same beneficial and adverse effects as another biologic drug (usually a branded, marketed product) but without identical structure.

bougie—A thick but somewhat flexible tapered tube that is used for **dilation** of a narrowed area of the **esophagus**, i.e., a **stricture** or a ring. They come in various sizes, and some can be inserted over a guide wire.

capsule endoscopy—Examination of part of the GI tract, usually the small intestine, using a capsule containing a camera, light source, battery, antenna, and transmitter. The capsule takes pictures and beams them to a receiver that the patient wears. The patient swallows the capsule with water, as if taking a large pill. The capsule is passed out into the stool and is not retrieved. Also known as wireless capsule endoscopy.

carbohydrate—1. A molecule composed of carbon, hydrogen, and oxygen. 2. A food containing sugars (**monosaccharides, disaccharides, oligosaccharides,** or **polysaccharides**). Carbohydrates are the major source of energy in the body.

carcinoembryonic antigen—A protein produced in the developing fetus and in some tumors, especially **colon** cancer. It may be useful in detecting recurrence of **colon** cancer after surgery. It is not a test for cancer in a healthy person.

cautery—1. Electric current, heat, or a chemical which destroys tissue for medical purposes. 2. Cauterization is the use of any of these modalities to destroy tissue.

C. Diff—See *Clostridium difficile.*

CEA—See **carcinoembryonic antigen.**

cecal intubation rate—The percentage of colonoscopies in which the **cecum** is reached.

cecum—1. The last part of the **colon** that the **scope** reaches during **colonoscopy**. 2. The first part of the **colon** that the intestinal contents reach after leaving the small intestine. It resembles a pouch and contains the appendix.

celiac disease—A disease in which gluten, a protein contained in wheat, rye, and barley, activates the immune system in the small intestine. The resulting inflammation may cause symptoms such as diarrhea, weight loss, or constipation; children may have failure to thrive. Some people have no symptoms. Longstanding active celiac disease is associated with **lymphoma**, a cancer of lymphatic tissue. Treatment is a **gluten-free diet.**

chemotherapy—Medications to treat cancer or chronic infections.

cholangitis—Inflammation or infection of the bile ducts. See also **sclerosing cholangitis**.

cholecystectomy—Surgical removal of the gallbladder.

cholecystitis—**Inflammation** of the gallbladder.

choledocholithiasis—A stone in the common bile duct.

cholelithiasis—A stone in the gallbladder; gallstones.

chromoendoscopy—A procedure in which the lining of the **colon** is sprayed with dye during colonoscopy, allowing better visualization of abnormal areas for **biopsy**. This technique allows better detection of **dysplasia**.

chronic—Long-lasting, persistent. **Hepatitis** is often diagnosed as chronic if it has been present for six months. In contrast to **acute,** which is of short duration.

cirrhosis—Abnormal scar tissue (**fibrosis**) in the liver which forms **nodules** and leads to impaired liver function. It is caused not only by alcohol but also hepatitis B, hepatitis C, **autoimmune hepatitis**, and other liver disorders.

clip—See **endoclip**.

Clostridium difficile (*C. difficile* or C-diff)—A bacteria that can be a minimal component of the normal stool bacteria. *Clostridium difficile* infection is associated with the use of antibiotics, especially when given in a hospital or nursing home. The antibiotics kill off many other competing bacteria, allowing the *Clostridium difficile* to overgrow and cause persistent diarrhea which is often difficult to treat. A serious **colitis**, known as **pseudomembranous colitis**, may result. *Clostridium difficile* is transmitted by **spores**, which may be unknowingly ingested.

colitis—**Inflammation** of the colon. See also **ulcerative colitis**.

colon—1. The part of the large intestine between the **cecum** and rectum, inclusive. It removes fluid, electrolytes, and some nutrients from the remnants of food which pass from the small intestine into the colon. 2. This term is often used synonymously with the large intestine.

colonoscopy—The insertion of a long **scope** by which the inside of the large intestine is viewed. **Polyps** can be removed, **biopsies** of normal or abnormal areas can be done, and bleeding can be treated.

colostomy—A surgically placed connection between the **colon** and the skin. The patient must wear a bag over the opening (**stoma**) to catch and release the fecal material. Although dreaded by many, patients adapt to this remarkably well, and the newer bags are easy to apply and remove.

Coumadin—See **warfarin**.

Crohn's disease—A disease of unknown cause which may cause mild, moderate, or severe inflammation in any part of the digestive tract. It may be an **autoimmune disease**. It typically affects the **terminal ileum**

(the last part of the small intestine) or the **colon** or both. It may be impossible to distinguish Crohn's disease from **ulcerative colitis**, but Crohn's disease often occurs in a pattern of abnormal areas separated by normal areas (skip areas) and affects all layers of the **colon** wall (**ulcerative colitis** almost always starts in the rectum and affects only the inner lining of the colon). Abdominal pain, diarrhea, weight loss, and, more rarely, bleeding are typical symptoms of Crohn's disease. Treatment is with anti-inflammatory or **immunosuppressive drugs** and **biologic drugs,** depending on the severity of the disease.

CT colonography—A **CT scan** of the colon, performed after a **colon** prep and oral contrast administration. Also known as virtual colonoscopy.

CT scan—computed tomographic scan; an imaging procedure using X-rays taken from a 360-degree angle around the patient. A computer integrates the results and produces excellent cross-sectional images of most internal organs. CT scans can lead to diagnosis of many gastrointestinal conditions, including cancer. Oral or **intravenous** contrast is often used to enhance the images. Radiation exposure is a concern, given the high frequency with which CT scans are done these days.

curative resection—Surgical removal of a portion of the **GI tract** with the intent to cure. The term is most commonly used regarding cancer.

deductible—A term used in the insurance industry to denote a dollar amount of medical bills that must be paid by the patient out of pocket before the insurance plan starts to pay anything. The deductible takes effect at the start of each calendar year. Higher deductibles should result in lower premiums (cost of the insurance). The deductible does not apply to all services. For example, the deductible should not apply to a screening **colonoscopy.**

deoxyribonucleic acid (DNA)—Material in cells of the body that comprises the **genes** (hereditary factors) that contain your biologic information and instruct your cells how to function. Most DNA is located in the nucleus of the cell. The DNA molecule contains a code which is the order of four nitrogen bases which keep repeating throughout the long molecule. Groups of these bases make **genes**. DNA can copy itself for cell division.

dermatitis herpetiformis—A rash consisting of bumps and blisters which can be itchy or burning. It is typically located on knees, elbows, back, or buttocks, and is the same on both sides. The rash can come and go. It is diagnosed with a skin biopsy. Dermatitis herpetiformis is strongly related to celiac disease and is not a herpes virus. It is treated with a gluten-free diet and sometimes with a medicine called dapsone.

diabetes mellitus—A group of diseases of the body's handling of blood glucose (sugar), resulting in elevated levels of glucose in the blood. Type 2 diabetes comprises 90 percent of cases and occurs when the pancreas does not make enough insulin or the cells of the body do not use insulin properly, a condition also known as insulin resistance (insulin regulates the blood glucose and allows cells to absorb glucose from the blood). Type 2 diabetes is caused mainly by obesity and inactivity. In type 1 diabetes, the pancreas makes little or no insulin.

dietary fiber—Substances in food from plants that are not digested. Includes soluble fiber, which consists of **carbohyrates** and will dissolve in water, and insoluble fiber, which does not dissolve in water.

dilation—A procedure in which a narrowed area of the **GI tract** is made wider. This is most commonly done in the **esophagus** for trouble swallowing, but it can be done in any part of the **GI tract**.

disaccharide—A sugar (**carbohydrate**) composed of two **monosaccharides**. Has two carbon rings. Examples: **lactose**, maltose, and sucrose.

distal—An area relatively far away from a specific point of reference. The opposite of **proximal**.

distal colon—1. The last part of the **colon** through which the stool passes. 2. The first part of the **colon** reached by the colonoscope. 3. The left colon.

diverticulitis—An infection or inflammation of a **diverticulum,** almost always in the colon. It causes pain, typically in the left lower abdomen in the United States. It is usually diagnosed with a **CT scan**. Antibiotics are usually needed, and hospitalization for **intravenous** antibiotic administration is often required. Complications include spontaneous **perforation** and **abscess** formation.

diverticulosis—The presence of numerous diverticula in the **colon** without infection or inflammation.

diverticulum—A pouch in the digestive tract caused by a defect in the underlying muscle layer. *Plural*: diverticula.

DNA—See deoxyribonucleic acid.

duodenum—The first part of the small intestine, immediately following the stomach.

dysplasia—Abnormal size, shape, or arrangement of cells which can be a forerunner of cancer. More severe dysplasia, known as high-grade dysplasia, has a higher risk of progression to cancer.

edema—Abnormal accumulation of fluid in a part of the body, commonly in the ankles or lower legs.

EGD—See **esophagogastroduodenoscopy**.

endoclip—A metal device which can be passed through an **endoscope** in order to close two surfaces. Endoclips, or clips, can be used to control GI bleeding or close potential or actual **perforations**.

endoscope—1. A flexible instrument used to visualize the inside of a hollow structure. 2. A **scope** to view the upper **GI tract**.

endoscopic mucosal resection—A method of removing an abnormal area in the lining of the GI tract, such as **Barrett's esophagus** with **dysplasia,** large or flat **polyps**, and some superficial tumors, using an **endoscope**. It involves raising the abnormality by injecting fluid under it and then removing the tissue with a snare wire or similar device. An **endoscopic ultrasound** can be done to assess the depth of the abnormality; if it is too deep, the procedure becomes too risky or technically difficult. Also known as EMR, endoscopic mucosal resection is an alternative to surgery for some disorders.

endoscopic retrograde cholangiopancreatography (ERCP)—An upper-GI endoscopy using a specially designed side-viewing scope, also known as a duodenoscope. The procedure can include injection of contrast into the biliary or pancreatic ducts for X-rays, performance of a **sphincterotomy**, insertion of instruments to remove gallstones, and placement of stents. The greatest risk of ERCP is pancreatitis, which can be severe.

endoscopic ultrasound—A procedure in which an endoscope with an ultrasound probe on the tip is inserted into the mouth or anus to perform an ultrasound from inside the body. Abbreviated as **EUS**. This allows a much more detailed view of certain structures. **EUS** may be used to diagnose esophageal cancer, pancreatic cysts and cancer, and rectal cancer. The depth of invasion and involvement of **lymph nodes** can be evaluated. Using a very thin needle, cells or fluid can be withdrawn (**fine-needle aspiration, or FNA**).

endoscopy—The examination of a hollow structure using an **endoscope**. Includes **EGD** and **colonoscopy**. Also used to denote visualization of the small intestine with a specialized capsule containing a camera, light source, battery, and transmitter (see **capsule endoscopy** and chapter 7, "Overview of Colon Cancer").

endoscopy technician ("tech")—Someone who has undergone training to assist with endoscopic procedures and maintain proper care of the equipment.

epinephrine—A drug that constricts blood vessels. It can be injected close to the source of GI bleeding. It will stop the bleeding and allow more precise determination of the exact site of the bleeding.

ERCP—See **endoscopic retrograde cholangiopancreatography.**

esophagogastroduodenoscopy—Examination of the upper-**GI tract**, e.g., the esophagus, stomach, and **duodenum**, with a flexible **endoscope**. Also known as **EGD**.

esophagus—A hollow cylindrical organ connecting the throat to the stomach.

ether—An inflammable liquid producing a vapor with a typical odor. It was first administered as an anesthetic by inhalation of the vapor in the 1840s. Its use in the United States continued through the early/mid-1900s, after which it was replaced by safer anesthetic agents.

ethylene glycol—A compound used as antifreeze, not to be confused with **polyethylene glycol**. Ethylene glycol is toxic to people.

EUS—See endoscopic ultrasound.

exocrine—a cell, **gland**, or organ that secretes a substance that it produces via a duct.

fatty liver—Accumulation of fat in the liver which is most commonly caused by alcohol use, **diabetes mellitus**, or being overweight. Liver enzymes may or may not be elevated. In some, it can progress to non-alcoholic steatohepatitis, a non-viral form of **hepatitis** in which inflammation is directed against the fat, or **cirrhosis**. Fatty liver has become so common due to the present obesity epidemic that a large increase in the incidence of **cirrhosis** is expected in 20–30 years.

fermentation—The breaking down of organic compounds to simpler substances, including liquids and gases, in the absence of oxygen.

ferritin—The storage form of iron. It can be measured in the blood. It is elevated in hereditary hemochromatosis but also in infection or inflammation.

fiber—See **dietary fiber**.

fibrosis—Scar tissue formed in the body in order to heal infection, inflammation, or injury. The fibrosis can be harmful if too extensive, as in **cirrhosis** of the liver.

fine-needle aspiration—The procedure in which a very thin needle is passed from an **endoscope** during **EUS**, through the wall of the intestine, and into a structure (examples are pancreas, pancreatic cyst, liver, or lymph node) in order to remove cells or fluid for analysis. Abbreviated **FNA**.

fistula—An abnormal connection (tunnel) between two organs or between one organ and the body surface.

fluoroscopy—Real-time imaging of structures inside the body by X-rays. Fluoroscopy is used in connection with some endoscopic techniques. There is radiation exposure to the patient with fluoroscopy.

FNA—See **fine-needle aspiration**.

FODMAP—1. Short-chain **carbohydrates** which are poorly absorbed and cause symptoms in people with irritable bowel syndrome. A low-FODMAP diet can be helpful. 2. Acronym for **fermentable oligosaccharides, disaccharides, monosaccharides**, and **polyols**.

functional—relating to how well an organ of the body works. An organ with a functional disorder may appear normal on visualization or biopsy, but may not work properly. Irritable bowel syndrome is an example.

gangrene—a form of tissue death and decay, associated with loss of blood supply. Bacterial infection often follows.

gastroenterology—The study of the normal function and disorders of the **GI tract**, including the liver, gallbladder, and pancreas.

gastroparesis—A disorder in which the stomach empties abnormally slowly. Food may stay in the stomach much longer than normal, and nausea and vomiting are common symptoms.

gene—The unit of heredity. Genes are composed of DNA in humans and in almost all living things. Genes can be passed to offspring and determine some of the characteristics of the offspring.

generic—Refers to a medication that can be made by many manufacturers. The patent on the original drug has expired, and the chemical name of the drug may be used by other manufacturers. Example: Omeprazole was originally marketed as Prilosce and was protected by patent and trademark laws. At this time, generic omeprazole is made by several companies.

genotype—1. Refers to either the entire genetic makeup of a person or organism, or one particular set of genes. 2. In hepatitis C virus infection, one of seven major strains of the virus. Genotype may influence disease progression and response to therapy.

GERD—**GE reflux** disease.

GE reflux—Gastroesophageal reflux. The backflow of stomach contents into the esophagus and sometimes the throat and respiratory tract. GE reflux often causes heartburn but may not have any symptoms. It may lead to esophageal **ulcers** or **strictures**, **Barrett's esophagus**, or esophageal cancer.

GI—Gastrointestinal.

GI tract—The long, tubular pathway from the mouth to the anus that is involved with the digestion of food and absorbing nourishment for the body. The GI tract includes the esophagus, stomach, small intestine, and large intestine. The liver, gallbladder, and pancreas, which are directly connected and provide substances needed for digestion, are also considered part of the GI tract.

gland—A group of cells or an organ that creates a chemical that is used for some function outside of the cell. The substance produced may be used elsewhere in the body or excreted from the body. Examples: pancreas, salivary glands, sweat glands. See **exocrine** gland.

gluten-free diet—A diet that does not contain wheat, rye, or barley. It is essential for the treatment of **celiac disease**. Oats are usually best avoided in a gluten-free diet, especially initially, because products made from oats are often contaminated with gluten during the manufacturing process. Certain brands of oats are free from contamination, but this needs to be carefully researched before ingesting.

H2 blocker—A group of drugs that reduce the output of stomach acid, also known as histamine H2 receptor antagonists. They are used to treat **GERD** and **ulcers**. They are less potent than **PPI** drugs but may be more effective at night. Examples: cimetidine, famotidine, nizatidine, and ranitidine.

HCV-RNA—1. The RNA, or ribonucleic acid, molecule that contains the genetic information of the hepatitis C virus. 2. A positive test for HCV-RNA indicates that the hepatitis C virus is actively reproducing. A negative test indicates that the hepatitis C virus infection is inactive or has been cured by antiviral treatment.

heater probe—A catheter which is passed through an **endoscope** and can deliver heat to a bleeding site. The heat disrupts tissue, including blood vessels, and promotes clotting. It is often used in combination with **epinephrine** injections to control **GI** bleeding.

Helicobacter pylori (*H. pylori*)—A bacterial species that lives in the stomach and can cause **ulcers** or inflammation of the stomach (gastritis).

hemorrhoid—Veins of the anus and rectum. They may be on the inside (internal) or outside (external). They are graded from 1 to 4, with grade 1 being the most minor. Most cause no symptoms, but they can cause pain, bleeding, itching, and other discomforts.

hemorrhoid banding—Placement of a rubber band around a portion of a **hemorrhoid**, in order to reduce bleeding or other symptoms. If the band is placed far enough inside, there will usually be no pain.

hepatic encephalopathy—A spectrum of impairments in mental status caused by cirrhosis of the liver. Hepatic encephalopathy can be clinically obvious (overt) or very subtle (covert). In either case, the diseased liver cannot inactivate certain toxic substances absorbed from the **GI tract**.

hepatitis—Inflammation of the liver. The term is commonly used to imply viral hepatitis (hepatitis A–E), but hepatitis can be non-viral, as in **autoimmune hepatitis**, the result of medications, **fatty liver**, or other disorders.

hernia—A loop of bowel that protrudes into a place where it should not be.

hiatus hernia—The protrusion of the stomach upward, through the esophageal hiatus (the normal opening in the diaphragm through which the esophagus passes) and into the chest.

HIDA scan—A nuclear medicine scan of the gallbladder. A substance is given intravenously which becomes concentrated in the gallbladder. Images are made, following which another substance, cholecystokinin, which normally causes the gallbladder to contract, may be given. The amount of gallbladder emptying can be determined from the images. HIDA stands for hepatobiliary iminodiacetic acid, a substance which is normally taken up by the liver and then added to the bile that travels to the gallbladder. The HIDA is linked to a radioactive marker that can be scanned in the nuclear medicine department.

high-fiber diet—A diet rich in whole grains, fruits, and vegetables that contain **dietary fiber**.

HIV—Human immunodeficiency virus, the cause of acquired immune deficiency syndrome (AIDS). HIV infection is often seen in the same patients who have hepatitis C.

hormone—A chemical substance produced by one type of body cell that travels via the blood to another organ or tissue where it exerts a specific effect.

hyperplastic—A type of growth that may be recognized as a **colon polyp**, in which the cells are increased but are normal in appearance and arrangement. Hyperplastic **polyps** in the **colon** have almost no risk of becoming cancer.

ileus—An impairment of the motility of the large or small intestine.

immunosuppressive drug—A medication that blocks the body's ability to react against infections or foreign substances.

incarcerated hernia—A **hernia** in which a loop of bowel has protruded into an area that it should not be and cannot be pushed back (reduced). Such a **hernia** can become strangulated; see **strangulated hernia**.

incidence—The frequency with which a new case of a certain condition will occur in a given time period; that is, the number of new cases of **colon** cancer diagnosed in a particular country in 2017 is the incidence of **colon** cancer in that country.

inflammation—A response of the body to injury or infection that intends to destroy or isolate the underlying cause or the damaged tissue. White blood cells are central in mediating this response. Inflammation typically results in warmth, redness, and swelling of the affected tissue. Pain and loss of function can result.

inguinal hernia—A **hernia** in the groin.

intravenous (IV)—Within a vein. Often refers to drugs or fluids administered into a vein.

intubation—1. The insertion of a tube or **scope** into a hollow organ or body cavity. 2. Cecal intubation refers to the tip of the **scope** reaching the **cecum**. 3. Commonly used to describe the insertion of a tube into the **trachea** to provide assistance with breathing or to protect the airway during **EGD** and removal of foreign bodies from the **esophagus** (otherwise, the foreign body could possibly be dropped into the airway; not a good result).

jaundice—A yellow discoloration of the whites of the eyes and the skin, caused by increased levels of bile pigments in the blood; seen in advanced liver disease or bile duct obstruction.

lactose—A sugar contained in milk and other dairy products. It is a **disaccharide** (has two carbon rings) and is broken down into glucose and galactose by the enzyme lactase.

lactose intolerance—A deficiency of lactase, which digests **lactose**. A common cause of diarrhea, gas, cramps, and nausea.

laparoscopy—A surgical procedure in which a scope is inserted through very small incisions to examine the abdominal organs.

laryngoscopy—Visualization of the back of the throat and vocal cords, generally done by an ear, nose, and throat physician. There are two methods. Indirect laryngoscopy uses a mirror inserted into the back of the throat. Direct laryngoscopy views through a very thin scope inserted through the mouth, or for very flexible scopes, through the nose.

legume—1. A plant with long pods containing seeds. 2. A food consisting of pods or seeds from such plants. Examples: beans, peas, lentils.

lower esophageal sphincter—The muscles in the distal esophagus that relax when food passes through and remain contracted at other times, preventing **reflux** of acid from the stomach into the esophagus. The lower esophageal sphincter is not a structure that is visualized during an **EGD**. It may malfunction in patients with **GERD**.

lumen—The opening within a hollow or tubular organ.

lymph node—Storage site for certain types of white blood cells involved in immunity; also functions as a filter for bacteria and foreign bodies. They're located throughout the body and are connected to each other and to the bloodstream by lymphatic vessels.

lymphocyte—A type of white blood cell that is important in protecting the body from infections or cancer cells.

lymphoma—Cancer of lymphoid tissue.

melena—Black tarry stool which denotes bleeding from the GI tract, most commonly from the **esophagus**, stomach, or **duodenum** (the upper **GI tract**).

metastasis—A cancer deposit in another organ not in direct contact with the origin of the cancer.

metastasize—To spread to another organ.

metastatic—Describes a cancer or other disease process that has spread to another organ to which it is not directly connected. Different types of cancer may preferentially spread to certain organs. **Colon** cancer most commonly **metastasizes** to the liver. The metastatic deposits are called metastases.

methylprednisolone—A strong anti-inflammatory medication in the corticosteroid family that is given intravenously in hospitalized patients with severe inflammatory bowel disease.

microbiome—All of the microorganisms that live on or in the human body. They may be bacteria, viruses, fungi, or parasites. The estimated number is up to 100 trillion, or ten times the number of cells that make up the body. In addition to the GI tract, they may live on the skin or in the mouth, nose, and vagina.

microbiota—See **microbiome**.

microscopic colitis—Inflammation of the **colon** in which the **colon** appears normal when viewed through the **scope**, but biopsies show increased numbers of certain white blood cells.

midazolam—A sedative drug used for GI procedures. It generally causes amnesia for the time when high levels are in the body. Versed is the brand name for midazolam, a member of the class of drugs known as **benzodiazepines**.

monoclonal antibody—A pure antibody derived from identical immune cells.

monosaccharide—The basic unit of sugars, or **carbohydrates**. Contains one carbon ring. Also known as simple sugars. Examples are galactose and glucose.

motility—Spontaneous movement, e.g., the contractions of the muscle of the GI tract that move the food particles along.

MRCP—Magnetic resonance cholangiopancreatography. A type of **MRI** that can visualize the biliary and pancreatic ducts.

MRI—Magnetic resonance imaging. An imaging technique using magnetic fields. An advantage to MRI is that it does not use radiation.

mutation—A change in the genetic material of an organism.

necrosis—The death of cells of a localized area of the body. For example, necrotizing pancreatitis is cell death in a part of the pancreas during severe acute pancreatitis.

neo-adjuvant chemotherapy—Medications used to treat cancer before surgery is done, in order to shrink the tumor and make the chances of completely removing the entire cancer more likely.

nodule—A solid, round portion of tissue which is demarcated in some way.

NSAID—Non-steroidal anti-inflammatory drug. Used for arthritis and other painful conditions. Examples are ibuprofen and naproxen. They may cause ulcers in the GI tract, especially in the stomach and duodenum.

nucleotide—A component of nucleic acid (DNA or RNA).

olestra—A fat substitute, also known as Olean, that contains no fat or calories. It lowers the fat content of high-fat foods such as potato chips. Side effects include cramps, gas, and loose stools. Olestra may interfere with the absorption of fat-soluble vitamins (A, D, E, and K). It can interfere with the function of the colonoscope.

oligosaccharide—A **carbohydrate** consisting of a small number of simple sugars, or **monosaccharides**.

orifice—The entrance or opening into a body cavity.

OSHA—Occupational Safety and Health Administration. A U.S. government agency under the Department of Labor concerned with safety in the workplace. It sets and enforces standards for safety. It is concerned with workplace violence, which could include verbal abuse.

osmosis—The passage of fluid through a membrane into an area with a higher concentration of particles. In irritable bowel syndrome, short-chain sugars (**FODMAPs**) remain in the bowel **lumen** in high concentration, and water migrates into the bowel by osmosis.

ostomy—An opening to the skin that is created surgically, as in **colostomy** or ileostomy.

palpitations—Heartbeats that can be felt. They can be fast or slow, regular or irregular.

papilla—The major papilla is area comprising the opening of the common bile duct and pancreatic duct into the duodenum and the muscle fibers (**sphincter of Oddi**) that regulate flow from these ducts into the duodenum. The minor papilla is the opening of the accessory pancreatic duct into the duodenum.

paracentesis—Removal of fluid, known as **ascites**, from the abdominal cavity.

pathologist—A physician who looks at tissue samples from patients, living or deceased, under a microscope. Pathologists also perform autopsies.

pepsin—An enzyme produced in the stomach that digests protein.

perforation—An opening or tear in any part of the GI tract that occurs as a result of a disease or as a complication of a procedure.

perianal—Near the anus. A common site of **fistulas** in **Crohn's disease**.

PET scan—See **positron emission tomography**.

pH—A measure of acidity.

pharynx—Throat.

phlebotomy—Removal of blood from the body, through a vein.

Plavix—A medication that reduces blood clotting by interfering with the action of platelets. The **generic** name is clopidogrel. It's used in patients with heart disease or stroke, for treatment or prevention of adverse events, including worsening of the underlying disease.

polyethylene glycol—A substance used in bowel preps. It is a large molecule that is not absorbed into the body after ingestion. Rather, it softens the stool by remaining in the gut and drawing water into the lumen.

polymorphism—1. Existing in several forms. 2. In hepatitis C virus infection, polymorphisms are small variations in the structure of the virus that may occur naturally or after antiviral treatment. Some polymorphisms are associated with resistance to certain antiviral drugs, and testing for them is necessary before using those drugs.

polyol—Although known as sugar alcohol, polyols are not sugars (not composed of **monosaccharides**) and do not have effects commonly associated with alcohol. Polyols are used in the food industry as low-calorie sugar replacements that do not cause tooth decay. Examples: isomalt, maltitol, sorbitol, xylitol.

polyp—An abnormal growth of tissue, commonly seen in the **colon** and stomach. GI tract polyps can be **benign** or malignant; **benign polyps** can be adenomatous or **hyperplastic** (see **adenoma** and **hyperplastic**). They can also occur in other parts of the body.

polypectomy—Removal of a **polyp** during an **endoscopy** or surgery.

polysaccharide—A complex sugar containing multiple **monosaccharides**. Examples: cellulose, glycogen, and starch.

portal hypertension—A rise in blood pressure in the system of blood vessels that transport blood and absorbed food particles from the small intestine to the liver.

portal vein—A large vein that receives blood leaving the spleen and GI tract. It brings nutrients that have been absorbed in the small intestine to the liver for processing. The portal vein transports 75 percent of the blood supply to the liver; the remainder comes from the hepatic artery.

positron emission tomography—An imaging procedure, commonly known as a PET scan. It measures the chemical (metabolic) activity of cells. It is useful in evaluating the response to cancer treatments.

potassium—A chemical element that has important functions within the cells of the body. It can be measured in the blood. Very high or low values can be extremely dangerous. Potassium levels can be greatly influenced by medications used to treat **ascites** and **edema**.

PPI—See **proton pump inhibitor**.

prednisone—A medication that suppresses inflammation. It is useful in **Crohn's disease** or **ulcerative colitis**, but serious side effects limit it to short-term use. It is also used in other **autoimmune diseases**, allergic conditions, and in transplant patients.

probiotic—Living microorganisms, usually bacteria or yeast, which are ingested in food or pills with the intention of achieving a health benefit.

propylene glycol—A compound used as antifreeze, not to be confused with **polyethylene glycol**. Propylene glycol is toxic in people.

proton pump inhibitor—Medications used to treat heartburn, reflux, and ulcers. Proton pump inhibitors, or **PPIs**, block the production of acid in the stomach. They do this by inactivating the pump in certain cells of the stomach that pump out hydrogen ions.

proximal—An area close to a specific point of reference. The proximal jejunum is the first area reached by digested food as it leaves the duodenum. Opposite of **distal**.

proximal colon—The right colon; the first part of the **colon** reached by the remnants of digested food, but the last part reached by the **scope**. See **distal colon**.

PSC—See **sclerosing cholangitis, primary**.

pseudocyst—A cyst-like structure without a true wall containing lining cells. A pseudocyst can be a complication of acute pancreatitis in which there is a collection of fluid, pancreatic enzymes, and tissue having undergone **necrosis**, surrounded by inflammation and scar tissue.

pseudomembranous colitis—Inflammation of the **colon** caused by Clostridium difficile, characterized by a pseudomembrane consisting of yellow to white material that appears to line the **colon** in some areas.

pylorus—The opening in the **distal** stomach that connects the stomach and the duodenum, the first part of the small intestine.

quasispecies—Multiple forms of the virus with small differences that exist simultaneously in patients with chronic hepatitis C. The quasispecies nature of the hepatitis C virus makes it difficult for the immune system to clear the virus and has so far prevented the development of an effective vaccine.

radiofrequency ablation—The deliverance of intense heat to a diseased area while leaving the surrounding area relatively unaffected. Used in **Barrett's esophagus** with **dysplasia** and small cancers in the esophagus and liver.

reflux—The situation when fluid in a hollow organ or vessel goes in the direction opposite that intended. See also **GE reflux**.

remission—Resolution or disappearance of symptoms. A remission can be partial or complete. In cancer, remission denotes the absence of any detectable cancer; cancer cells could still be present but in numbers below the detection limit of tests such as **CT scan**.

renal—Pertaining to the kidneys.

ribavirin—An antiviral drug used in the treatment of hepatitis C virus infection, in combination with other drugs. It can cause severe anemia.

Schatski ring—A smooth, thin structure in the lower (**distal**) **esophagus** that can narrow the **lumen**, leading to trouble swallowing solid foods.

sclerosing cholangitis, primary—A disorder of the bile ducts characterized by narrowed and dilated areas of bile ducts within or outside the liver. It is associated with **ulcerative colitis**. There is no effective treatment, and it can be complicated by cancers, including cholangiocarcinoma, a cancer of the bile ducts with an extremely poor prognosis. Abbreviated **PSC**.

scope—Abbreviation for colonoscope or **endoscope**.

snare and cautery—A method of **polyp** removal in which a wire loop is placed around the **polyp** and tightened, and then an electric current is passed through the wire loop. The combination of pressure from the wire loop and electric current cuts the **polyp**, and once separated from the wall of the **GI tract**, it can be suctioned through the **scope** or removed along with the **scope**.

sphincter of Oddi—The muscle fibers surrounding the merged bile and pancreatic ducts at the point where the ducts reach the duodenum, at the

ampulla of Vater. The sphincter of Oddi regulates the flow of bile and pancreatic enzymes into the duodenum and prevents backflow of partially digested food from the duodenum into the bile duct system.

sphincterotomy—1. Incision of a sphincter. 2. An incision of the **sphincter of Oddi** in order to facilitate the removal of bile duct stones and allow better drainage of bile.

spider vein—An abnormal blood vessel with tiny branches coming out from a central point, resembling a spider. Seen in **cirrhosis** of the liver and pregnancy. Also known as spider angioma.

spontaneous bacterial peritonitis—An infection of **ascites** in patients with **cirrhosis** that has no surgically correctable source.

spore—An inactive, non-reproductive form of a bacteria which can later germinate and cause active infection. Similar to a seed. Spores are resistant to many environmental changes. *Clostridium difficile* infection is transmitted by spores.

squamous cell carcinoma—A cancer arising from and consisting of squamous cells, which are cells of the skin or cells resembling those of the skin which line internal organs. Squamous cell carcinoma is one of the two major types of esophageal cancer. Many small skin cancers are squamous cell carcinomas and can be readily removed by a dermatologist.

stent—A device used to keep a hollow structure open. Can be placed inside a part of the **GI tract** or inside a blood vessel to bypass an obstruction.

stoma—An artificial opening between a hollow organ and the outside. In **gastroenterology**, refers to a loop of bowel which has been surgically connected to the skin, often in order to bypass an obstruction. See **colostomy**.

strain—A subtype of a bacteria or virus.

strangulated hernia—An **incarcerated hernia** in which a loop of bowel is constricted such that the blood supply is compromised, resulting in tissue damage. A strangulated **hernia** is an emergency and requires surgery.

stricture—A narrowing in the **GI tract**. Can also be seen in the ducts connecting the liver and pancreas to the small intestine. A stricture can lead to adverse consequences for the patient or may be silent.

suppository—A soft, gel-like medication, normally inserted into the anus. Suppositories are sometimes used in **ulcerative colitis**, limited to the rectum or recto-sigmoid.

surveillance colonoscopy—A colonoscopy done at regular intervals for monitoring of **Crohn's disease** or **ulcerative colitis**. Biopsies are done to look for **dysplasia**. This term also refers to colonoscopies done at specified intervals after the removal of **adenomatous polyps** or colon cancer.

targeted therapy—Anti-cancer drugs that target specific molecules that influence cancer cell growth, progression, and spread. These drugs focus on that which makes cancer cells different from normal ones. Targeted therapies differ from chemotherapy, which attacks dividing cells in cancer and normal tissues. Targeted therapy and cancer may function well together.

tenesmus—Painful straining at stool. Tenesmus can be a sign of **ulcerative colitis** or rectal cancer. Similar to urgency, in which a person feels that they will have an accident if they do not reach a bathroom.

terminal ileum—The last part of the small intestine. It connects to the large intestine at the **cecum**.

time out—A protocol in which, just before a procedure, a checklist is reviewed. The time out includes such items as the patient's name, date of birth, allergies, type of procedure, which side of the patient will be operated on (if applicable), the name of the doctor, the specific instruments to be used, etc. It contributes significantly to patient safety.

TIPS—See **transjugular intrahepatic portosystemic shunt**.

TIVA—Total IV anesthesia.

toxic megacolon—Severe **dilation** of the **colon** in a critically ill patient. May be life-threatening. Can occur with **ulcerative colitis** and *Clostridium difficile* infection.

toxin—A substance produced by bacteria, plants, or animals that injures cells and causes disease. *Clostridium difficile* causes disease by producing a toxin.

trachea—A rigid hollow structure that connects the throat to the bronchial tubes that enter the lungs. Known as the windpipe.

transillumination—The appearance on the abdominal wall of the light from the tip of the colonoscope. This can help determine how far the scope has advanced. Pressure on the abdominal wall can enhance the visibility of the light.

transjugular intrahepatic portosystemic shunt (TIPS)—A hollow tube used in **portal hypertension** with **ascites** or esophageal **varices,** to connect, within the liver, an incoming portal vein and an outgoing hepatic vein. The TIPS reduces the portal pressure, often with significant improvement in **ascites** or **varices**. **Hepatic encephalopathy** can be made worse with TIPS.

triticale—A hybrid grain from wheat and rye. Triticale may be an unrecognized source of gluten (see **gluten-free diet**).

tumor necrosis factor (TNF)—A protein that has a key role in activating the immune system and stimulating inflammation. It also causes fever and death of tumor cells, among many other effects. Blockers of TNF (TNF inhibitors) reduce inflammation and are very useful in **Crohn's disease** and **ulcerative colitis**.

type 2 diabetes—See **diabetes mellitus**.

ulcer—A disruption of the lining of any part of the **GI tract**. Ulcers may have no symptoms but can cause pain, bleeding, or **perforation**.

ulcerative colitis—A disease of unknown cause that causes inflammation in some or all of the colon, starting in the rectum and extending a variable length without interruption. Diarrhea, urgency, and bleeding are typical symptoms. Ulcerative colitis may be difficult to distinguish from **Crohn's disease**. Treatment is with anti-inflammatory or **immunosuppressive drugs** and **biologic drugs**.

unresectable—A cancer that cannot be cured surgically.

varices—Dilated veins. In the **GI tract**, varices are seen in the **esophagus** or upper stomach, usually as a result of **cirrhosis** of the liver. They can occasionally be seen in the **duodenum** and rectum.

villi—Tiny projections covering the surface of the small intestine, greatly increasing its surface area and allowing for absorption of nutrients and fluids. Singular is villus.

villous adenoma—A **benign** but high-risk type of **colon polyp**. Villous adenomas have a growth pattern resembling projections that are stretched; it is sometimes described as cauliflower-like. They may produce increased amounts of mucus. They are often larger and have an increased risk of becoming cancer compared with tubular adenomas, the more common type. Patients with villous adenomas require more frequent **surveillance colonoscopies**.

virtual colonoscopy—See **CT colonography**.

warfarin—A medication that decreases blood clotting, i.e., an **anticoagulant**. It is used in many heart conditions or after strokes. It can be life-saving but carries a risk of potentially serious bleeding. **Coumadin** is a common brand name for warfarin.

Bibliography

AASLD-IDSA. "HCV Testing and Linkage to Care. Recommendations for Testing, Managing, and Treating Hepatitis C," http://www.hcvguidelines.org/full-report/ hcv-testing-and-linkage-care.

AASLD-IDSA. "Monitoring Patients Who Are Starting Hepatitis C Treatment, Are on Treatment, or Who Have Completed Therapy. Recommendations for Testing, Managing, and Treating Hepatitis C," http://hcvguidelines.org/full-report/monitor ing-patients-who-are-starting-hepatitis-c-treatment-are-treatment-or-have.

AASLD-IDSA. "Recommendations for Testing, Managing, and Treating Hepatitis C," http://hcvguidelines.org/.

AASLD-IDSA. "When and in Whom to Initiate HCV Therapy. Recommendations for Testing, Managing, and Treating Hepatitis C," http://hcvguidelines.org/full-report/ when-and-whom-initiate-hcv-therapy.

Afdhal, Nezam, Stephen Zeuzem, Paul Kwo, et al. "Ledipasvir and Sofosbuvir for Untreated HCV Genotype 1 Infection." *New England Journal of Medicine* 370, no. 20 (2014): 1889–98.

Agrawal, Sangeeta, Anand Bhupinderjit, Manoop S. Bhutani, et al. "Colorectal Cancer in African Americans." *American Journal of Gastroenterology* 100 (2005): 515–23.

Allergan.com. "Full Prescribing Information for Viberzi (Eluxadoline) Tablets for Oral Use," May 2015, https://www.allergan.com/assets/pdf/viberzi_pi.

American Cancer Society. "Cancer Facts and Figures 2016," 2016, www.cancer.org/ acs/groups/content/@research/documents/document/acspc-047079.pdf.

American Cancer Society. "How Is Cancer of the Esophagus Staged?" last updated February 4, 2016, http://www.cancer.org/cancer/esophaguscancer/detailedguide/ esophagus-cancer-staging.

American College of Gastroenterology. "Acid Reflux," http://patients.gi.org/topics/ acid-reflux/.

American Heart Association, "Added Sugars," http://www.heart.org/HEARTORG/HealthyLiving/HealthyEating/HealthyDietGoals/Added-Sugars_UCM_305858_Article.jsp#.V2a6t6L3hbw.

American Heart Association. "Know Your Fats," April 21, 2014, http://www.heart.org/HEARTORG/Conditions/Cholesterol/PreventionTreatmentofHighCholesterol/Know-Your-Fats_UCM_305628_Article.jsp#.V2YW_qL3hbw.

American Heart Association. "Saturated Fats," http://www.heart.org/HEARTORG/HealthyLiving/HealthyEating/Nutrition/Saturated-Fats_UCM_301110_Article.jsp#.V2ap-6L3hbx.

American Heart Association. "Trans Fats." Dallas: American Heart Association, http://www.heart.org/HEARTORG/HealthyLiving/FatsAndOils/Fats101/Trans-Fats_UCM_301120_Article.jsp#.V374ZqL3hbw.

Amri, Ramzi, Liliana G. Bordeianou, Patricia Sylla, and David L. Berger. "Impact of Screening Colonoscopy on Outcomes in Colon Cancer Surgery." *JAMA Surgery* 148 (2013): 747–54.

Angeli, Paolo, and Pere Gines. "Hepatorenal Syndrome, MELD Score, and Liver Transplantation: An Evolving Issue with Relevant Implications for Clinical Practice." *Journal of Hepatology* 57 (2012): 1135–40.

Anonymous. "Gut Health," http://www.healthknot.com/gut_health.html.

Antoniou, Tony, Erin M. Macdonald, Simon Hollands, et al. "Proton Pump Inhibitors and the Risk of Acute Kidney Injury in Older Patients: A Population-Based Cohort Study." *CMAJ Open* 3, no. 2 (2015): E166–71.

ASGE Standards of Practice Committee. "Complications of Colonoscopy." *Gastrointestinal Endoscopy* 74, no. 4 (2011): 745–52.

ASGE Standards of Practice Committee. "The Role of Endoscopy in Inflammatory Bowel Disease." *Gastrointestinal Endoscopy* 81, no. 5 (2015): 1101–21.

Associated Press. "Jackson's Death Officially Ruled a Homicide." *Today*, August 28, 2009, http://www.today.com/id/32598793/ns/today-today_entertainment/t/jacksons-death-officially-ruled-homicide/#.V2lVuqL3hbw.

Avila, Jim, and Christina Ng. "Michael Jackson's Doctor Guilty." *ABC News*, November 7, 2011, http://abcnews.go.com/US/michael-jacksons-doctor-guilty/story?id=14880567.

Bagdasarian, Natasha, Krishna Rao, and Preeti N. Malani. "Diagnosis and Treatment of *Clostridium difficile* in Adults: A Systematic Review." *JAMA* 313, no. 4 (2015): 398–408.

Balistreri, William F. "Should We All Go Gluten-Free?" *Medscape*, February 4, 2016, http://www.medscape.com/viewarticle/857971.

Banks, Peter A., Thomas I. Bollen, Christos Dervenis, et al. "Classification of Acute Pancreatitis—2012: Revision of the Atlanta Classification and Definitions by International Consensus." *Gut* 62 (2013): 102–11.

Barn Owl Conservation Network. "The Barn Owl's Sense of Hearing," http://www.bocn.org/factfile_detail.asp?id=39.

Barua, Soumitri, Robert Greenwald, Jason Grebely, Gregory Dore, Tracy Swan, and Lynn E. Taylor. "Restrictions for Medicaid Reimbursement of Sofosbuvir for the

Treatment of Hepatitis C Virus Infection in the United States." *Annals of Internal Medicine* 163, no. 3 (2015): 215–23.

Bedossa, Pierre, Thierry Poynard, and the METAVIR Cooperative Study Group. "An Algorithm for the Grading of Activity in Chronic Hepatitis C." *Hepatology* 23, no. 8 (1996): 289–93.

Bischoff, Stephan C. "Gut Health: A New Objective in Medicine?" *BMC Medicine* 9 (2011): 24, http://www.ncbi.nlm.nih.gov/pmc/articles/PMC3065426/.

Bouvard, Véronique, Dana Loomis, Kathryn Z. Guyton, et al. "Carcinogenicity of Consumption of Red and Processed Meat." *Lancet Oncology* 16 (2015): 1599–1600.

Brisebois, Elaine. "Steal This! The 4 R's of Healthy Digestion," March 28, 2013. http://www.elainebrisebois.com/the-4-rs-of-healthy-digestion/.

Brooks, Megan. "FDA Clears Obeticholic Acid for Primary Biliary Cholangitis." *Medscape*, May 31, 2016, http://www.medscape.com/viewarticle/864052.

Cafasso, Danielle E., and Richard R. Smith. "Symptomatic Cholelithiasis and Functional Disorders of the Biliary Tract." *Surgical Clinics of North America* 94 (2014): 233–56.

Canary, Lauren, R., Monina Klevens, and Scott D. Holmberg. "Limited Access to New Hepatitis C Virus Treatment under State Medicaid Programs." *Annals of Internal Medicine* 163, no. 3 (2015): 226–28.

Canto, Marcia Irene, Femme Harinck, Ralph H. Hruban, et al. "International Cancer of the Pancreas Screening (CAPS) Consortium Summit on the Management of Patients with Increased Risk for Familial Pancreatic Cancer." *Gut* 62 (2013): 339–47.

C Diff Foundation. "C. difficile Care at Home," https://cdifffoundation.org/2014/08/14/c-difficile-care-at-home/.

Centers for Disease Control and Prevention. "Epidemiology of the IBD," last updated March 31, 2015, http://www.cdc.gov/ibd/ibd-epidemiology.htm.

Centers for Disease Control and Prevention. "Hepatitis C: Testing Baby Boomers Saves Lives," May 2013, http://www.cdc.gov/feature/vitalsigns/hepatitis/.

Center for Medicaid and CHIP Services. "Assuring Medicaid Beneficiaries Access to Hepatitis C (HCV) Drugs," November 5, 2015, https://www.medicaid.gov/Medicaid-CHIP-Program-Information/By-Topics/Benefits/Prescription-Drugs/Downloads/Rx-Releases/State-Releases/state-rel-172.pdf.

Chopra, Sanjiv. "Patient Information: Cirrhosis (Beyond the Basics)." *UptoDate,* https://www.uptodate.com/contents/cirrhosis-beyond-the-basics?source=see_link.

Christensen, Jen. "New U.S. Dietary Guidelines Limit Sugar, Rethink Cholesterol." *CNN*, January 7, 2016, http://www.cnn.com/2016/01/07/health/2015-dietary-guidelines/index.html.

Cicero, Theodore J., Matthew S. Ellis, Hilary L. Surratt, and Stephen P. Kurtz. "The Changing Face of Heroin Use in the United States: A Retrospective Analysis of the Past 50 Years." *JAMA Psychiatry* 71, no. 7 (2014): 821–26.

Cleveland Clinic. "An Overview of Colorectal Cancer: Signs, Symptoms, and Stages," last modified October 29, 2013, http://my.clevelandclinic.org/health/diseases_conditions/hic-colorectal-cancer.

Cominelli, Fabio. "Inhibition of Leukocyte Trafficking in Inflammatory Bowel Disease." *New England Journal of Medicine* 369, no. 8 (2013): 775–76.

Corley, D. A., C. D. Jensen, A. R. Marks, et al. "Adenoma Detection Rate and the Risk of Colorectal Cancer and Death." *New England Journal of Medicine* 370 (2014): 1298–1306.

Corpechot, Christopher. "Primary Biliary Cirrhosis beyond Ursodeoxycholic Acid." *Seminars in Liver Disease* 36 (2016): 15–26.

Cotton, Peter, Grace H. Elta, C. Ross Carter, et al. "Gallbladder and Sphincter of Oddi Disorders." *Gastroenterology* 150, no. 6 (2016): 1420–29.

Denniston, Maxine M., Ruth B. Jiles, Jan Drobeniuc, et al. "Chronic Hepatitis C Virus Infection in the United States, National Health and Nutrition Examination Survey 2003 to 2010." *Annals of Internal Medicine* 160, no. 5 (2014): 293–300.

Desai, Tusar K., Veslav Stecevic, Chung-Ho Chang, Neal S. Goldstein, Kamran Badizadegan, and Glenn T. Furuta. "Association of Eosinophilic Inflammation with Esophageal Food Impaction in Adults." *Gastrointestinal Endoscopy* 61, no. 7 (2005): 795–801.

DeSalvo, Karen B., Richard Olsen, and Kellie O. Casavale. "Dietary Guidelines for Americans." *JAMA* 315, no. 5 (2016): 457–58.

Duke, Alan. "Joan Rivers Died from 'Therapeutic Complications,' Medical Examiner Says." *CNN*, October 16, 2014, http://www.cnn.com/2014/10/16/showbiz/joan -rivers-cause-of-death/index.html.

Dunavan, Jennifer. "Reading Gluten-Free Labels." *Fremont Tribune*, March 17, 2015, http://fremonttribune.com/lifestyles/food-and-cooking/reading-gluten-free-labels/ article_35a29a3d-a0dd-5917-bb88-ff9fc09a738b.html.

Elsagher, Brenda. *I'd Like to Buy a Bowel, Please*. Expert Publishing, 2006.

Elsagher, Brenda. *It's in the Bag and Under the Covers*. Expert Publishing, 2011.

El-Serag, Hashem B. "Hepatocellular Carcinoma." *New England Journal of Medicine* 365, no. 12 (2011): 1118–27.

Engel, Lawrence S., Wong-Ho Chow, Thomas L. Vaughan, et al. "Population Attrib-utable Risks of Esophageal and Gastric Cancers." *Journal of the National Cancer Institute* 95, no. 18 (2003): 1404–13.

Epstein, Lauren, Jennifer C. Hunter, M. Allison Arwady, et al. "New Delhi Metallo-β-Lactamase-Producing Carbapenem-Resistant *Escherichia coli* Associated with Exposure to Duodenoscopes." *JAMA* 312, no. 14 (2014): 1447–55.

Eswaran, Shanti, Jane Muir, and William D. Chey. "Fiber and Functional Gastrointes-tinal Disorders." *American Journal of Gastroenterology* 108, no. 5 (2013): 718–27.

Farci, Patrizia, and Robert H. Purcell. "Clinical Significance of Hepatitis C Virus Genotypes and Quasispecies." *Seminars in Liver Disease* 20 (2000): 103–26.

FDA. "FDA Approves Inflectra, a Biosimilar to Remicade," April 5, 2016, http://www .fda.gov/NewsEvents/Newsroom/PressAnnouncements/ucm494227.htm.

Feagan, Brian G., Paul Rutgeerts, Bruce E. Sands, et al. "Vedolizumab as Induction and Maintenance Therapy for Ulcerative Colitis." *New England Journal of Medi-cine* 369, no. 8 (2013): 699–710.

Ferenci, Peter, Alan Lockwood, Kevin Mullen, Ralph Tarter, Karin Weissenborn, An-dres T. Blei, and Members of the Working Party. "Hepatic Encephalopathy—Defi-nition, Nomenclature, Diagnosis, and Quantification: Final Report of the Working

Party at the 11th World Congress of Gastroenterology, Vienna, 1998." *Hepatology* 35, no. 3 (2002): 716–21.

Ferrarese, Alberto, Alberto Zanetto, Martina Gambato, et al. "Liver Transplantation for Viral Hepatitis in 2015." *World Journal of Gastroenterology* 22, no. 4 (2016): 1570–81.

Floch, Martin H. "Probiotics and Prebiotics." *Gastroenterology & Hepatology* 10, no. 10 (2014): 680–81.

Ford, Alexander C., Paul Moayyedi, Brian E. Lacy, et al. "American College of Gastroenterology Monograph on the Management of Irritable Bowel Syndrome and Chronic Idiopathic Constipation." *American Journal of Gastroenterology* 109, supplement 1 (2014): S2–S26.

Fox, Maggie. "Who's Mad about the New Dietary Guidelines? Cancer Experts, for One." *NBC News*, January 7, 2016, http://www.nbcnews.com/health/health-news/who-s-mad-about-new-dietary-guidelines-cancer-experts-one-n492026.

Furuta, Glenn T., and David A. Katzka. "Eosinophilic Esophagitis." *New England Journal of Medicine* 373 (2015): 1640–48.

Gabrielli, C., A. Zannini, R. Corradini, and S. Gafa. "Spread of Hepatitis C Virus Among Sexual Partners of HCVAb positive intravenous drug users. *Journal of Infection* 29 (1994): 17–22.

Getz, Lindsey. "Gluten-Free Fast Food—May I Take Your Order Please?" *Today's Dietitian* 16, no. 8 (2014): 28, http://www.todaysdietitian.com/newarchives/080114p28.shtml.

Gibson, Peter R., and Susan J. Shepherd. "Evidence-Based Dietary Management of Functional Gastrointestinal Symptoms: The FODMAP Approach." *Journal of Gastroenterology and Hepatology* 25 (2010): 252–58.

Gluten-Free Living, "Eating at Restaurants," June 12, 2013, http://www.glutenfreeliving.com/gluten-free-foods/gluten-free-eating-out/eating-at-restaurants/.

Goldstein, Michael J., and Edith Peterson Mitchell. "Carcinoembryonic Antigen in the Staging and Follow-up of Colorectal Cancer." *Cancer Investigation* 23, no. 4 (2005): 338–51.

Gomm, Willy, Klaus von Holt, Friederike Thomé, et al. "Association of Proton Pump Inhibitors with Risk of Dementia: A Pharmacoepidemiological Claims Data Analysis." *JAMA Neurology* 73, no. 4 (2016): 410–16.

Gottlieb, Jeff. "Michael Jackson Had Several Drugs in His System When He Died." *Los Angeles Times*, May 7, 2013, http://articles.latimes.com/2013/may/07/local/la-me-jackson-trial-20130507.

Haenisch, Britta, Klaus von Holt, Birgitt Wiese, et al. "Risk of Dementia in Elderly Patients with the Use of Proton Pump Inhibitors." *European Archives of Psychiatry and Clinical Neuroscience* 265, no. 5 (2015): 419–28.

Halmos, Emma P., Victoria A. Power, Susan J. Shepherd, Peter R. Gibson, and Jane G. Muir. "A Diet Low in FODMAPs Reduces Symptoms of Irritable Bowel Syndrome." *Gastroenterology* 146, no. 1 (2014): 67–75.

Hamburg, Margaret A. "Remarks of the Proposed Updates to the Nutrition Facts Label." U.S. Food and Drug Administration, February 27, 2014, http://www.fda.gov/newsevents/speeches/ucm387589.htm.

Hartocollis, Anemona. "Joan Rivers Died from Complication in Treatment, Officials Say." *New York Times*, October 16, 2014, http://www.nytimes.com/2014/10/17/nyre gion/joan-rivers-died-of-complication-in-treatment-medical-examiner-says.html.

Hasler, William L. "Physiology of Gastric Motility and Gastric Emptying." In *Textbook of Gastroenterology, Fourth Edition*, edited by Tadataka Yamada, 195–219. Philadelphia: Lippincott Williams & Wilkins, 2003.

Hayward, Kelly L., Elizabeth E. Powell, Katharine M. Irvine, and Jennifer H. Martin. "Can Paracetamol (Acetaminophen) Be Administered to Patients with Liver Impairment?" *British Journal of Clinical Pharmacology* 81, no. 2 (2015): 210–22.

Higdon, Jane, and Victoria J. Drake. "Fiber." Corvallis, Oregon: Linus Pauling Institute, Oregon State University, http://lpi.oregonstate.edu/mic/other-nutrients/fiber.

Hutchinson, S. J., S. M. Bird, and D. J. Goldberg. "Influence of Alcohol on the Progression of Hepatitis C Virus Infection: A Meta-analysis." *Clinical Gastroenterology and Hepatology* 3 (2005): 1150–59.

International Agency for Research on Cancer, World Health Organization. "IARC Monographs Evaluate Consumption of Red Meat and Processed Meat." International Agency for Research on Cancer, October 26, 2015, http://www.iarc.fr/en/media-centre/pr/2015/pdfs/pr240_E.pdf.

Italiano, Laura, and Julia Marsh. "Unplanned Biopsy Led to Joan Rivers' Death." *Page Six*, September 10, 2014, http://pagesix.com/2014/09/10/unplanned-biopsy-led-to-joan-rivers-death/.

Jackman, Tom. "Anesthesiologist Trashes Sedated Patient—And It Ends Up Costing Her." *Washington Post*, June 23, 2015, https://www.washingtonpost.com/local/anesthesiologist-trashes-sedated-patient-jury-orders-her-to-pay-500000/2015/06/23/cae05c00-18f3-11e5-ab92-c75ae6ab94b5_story.html?postshare=31814351 22381625.

Jones, Christopher M., Melinda Campopiano, Grant Baldwin, and Elinore McCance-Katz. "National and State Treatment Need and Capacity for Opioid Agonist Medication-Assisted Treatment." *American Journal of Public Health* 105, no. 8 (2015): e55–e63.

Kachaamy, Toufic, and Jasmohan S. Bajaj. "Diet and Cognition in Chronic Liver Disease." *Current Opinion in Gastroenterology* 27, (2011): 174–79.

Kahi, Charles J., Joseph C. Anderson, and Douglas K. Rex. "Screening and Surveillance for Colorectal Cancer: State of the Art." *Gastrointestinal Endoscopy* 77, no. 3 (2013): 335–50.

Kahi, Charles J., C. Richard Boland, Jason A. Dominitz, et al. "Colonoscopy Surveillance after Colorectal Cancer Resection: Recommendations of the US Multi-Society Task Force on Colon Cancer." *Gastrointestinal Endoscopy* 83, no. 3 (2016): 489–98.

Kamath, Patrick S., John J. Poterucha, and Jurgen Ludwig. "Primary Biliary Cirrhosis by Another Name Is Still PBC." *Journal of Hepatology* 63 (2015): 1066–77.

Katz, Mitchell H. "Failing the Acid Test: Benefits of Proton Pump Inhibitors May Not Justify the Risks for Many Users." *Archives of Internal Medicine* 170, no. 9 (2010): 747–78.

Kawaguchi, Takumi, Namiki Izumi, Michael R. Charlton, et al. "Branched-Chain Amino Acids as Pharmacological Nutrients in Chronic Liver Disease." *Hepatology* 54, no. 3 (2011): 1063–70.

Kelly, Ciarán P., and Melinda Dennis. "Patient Information: Celiac Disease in Adults (Beyond the Basics)." *UpToDate*, last modified November 12, 2015, https://www.uptodate.com/contents/celiac-disease-in-adults-beyond-the-basics?source=search_result&search=celiac+disease+patient+info&selectedTitle=3~150.

Kim, Stephen, Dana Russell, Mehdi Mohamadnejad, et al. "Risk Factors Associated with the Transmission of Carbapenem-Resistant Enterobacteriaceae via Contaminated Duodenoscopes." *Gastrointestinal Endoscopy* 83, no. 6 (2016): 1121–29.

Kovaleva, Julia, Frans T. M. Peters, Henry C. van der Mei, et al. "Transmission of Infection by Flexible Gastrointestinal Endoscopy and Bronchoscopy." *Clinical Microbiology Reviews* 26, no. 2 (2013): 231–54.

Kresser, Chris. "9 Steps to Perfect Health—#5: Heal Your Gut," February 24, 2011, http://chriskresser.com/9-steps-to-perfect-health-5-heal-your-gut/.

Kuller, Lewis H. "Do Proton Pump Inhibitors Increase the Risk of Dementia?" *JAMA Neurology* 73, no. 4 (2016): 379–81.

Kvasnovsky, C. L., S. Papagrigoriadis, and I. Bjarnason. "Increased Diverticular Complications with Nonsteroidal Anti-Inflammatory Drugs and Other Medications: A Systematic Review and Meta-analysis." *Colorectal Disease* 16, no. 6 (2014): O189–96.

Laine, Loren, Tonya Kaltenbach, Alan Barkun, et al. "SCENIC International Consensus Statement on Surveillance and Management of Dysplasia in Inflammatory Bowel Disease." *Gastroenterology* 148, no. 3 (2015): 639–51.

Lauridsen, Mette M., Leroy R. Thacker, Melanie B. White, et al. "In Patients with Cirrhosis, Driving Simulator Performance Is Associated with Real-Life Driving." *Clinical Gastroenterology and Hepatology* 14 (2016): 747–52.

Lazarus, Benjamin, Yuan Chen, Francis P. Wilson, et al. "Proton Pump Inhibitor Use and the Risk of Chronic Kidney Disease." *JAMA Internal Medicine* 176, no. 2 (2016): 238–46.

Lee, Christine H., Theodore Steiner, Elaine O. Petrof, et al. "Frozen vs Fresh Fecal Microbiota Transplantation and Clinical Resolution of Diarrhea in Patients with Recurrent *Clostridium difficile* Infection." *JAMA* 315, no. 2 (2016): 142–49.

Leffler, Daniel A., and J. Thomas Lamont. "*Clostridium difficile* Infection." *New England Journal of Medicine* 372, no. 16 (2015): 1539–48.

Leidner, Andrew J., Harrell W. Chesson, Fujie Xu, John W. Ward, Philip R. Spradling, and Scott D. Holmberg. "Cost-Effectiveness of Hepatitis C Treatment for Patients in Early Stages of Liver Disease." *Hepatology* 61, no. 6 (2015): 1860–69.

Lessa, Fernanda C., Yi Mu, Wendy C. Bamberg, et al. "Burden of *Clostridium difficile* Infection in the United States." *New England Journal of Medicine* 372, no. 9 (2015): 825–34.

Leung, Wesley, and Florence Wong. "Medical Management of Ascites." *Expert Opinion in Pharmacotherapy* 12, no. 8 (2011): 1269–83.

Lieberman, David A., Douglas K. Rex, Sidney J. Winawer, Frances M. Giardiello, David A. Johnson, and Theodore R. Levin. "Guidelines for Colonoscopy Surveillance after Screening and Polypectomy: A Consensus Update by the US Multi-Society Task Force on Colorectal Cancer." *Gastroenterology* 143, no. 9 (2012): 844–57.

Lobatón, T., S. Vermeire, G. Van Assche, and P. Rutgeerts. "Review Article: Anti-Adhesion Therapies for Inflammatory Bowel Disease." *Alimentary Pharmacology and Therapeutics* 39 (2014): 579–94.

Lowes, Robert. "FDA OKs *Epclusa*, First Drug for All Major Forms of HCV." *Medscape*, June 28, 2016, http://www.medscape.com/viewarticle/865487.

Manos, M. Michele, Valentina A. Shvachko, Rosemary C. Murphy, Jean Marie Arduino, and Norah J. Shire. "Distribution of Hepatitis C Virus Genotypes in a Diverse US Integrated Health Care Population." *Journal of Medical Virology* 84 (2012): 1744–50.

Marcus, Stephanie. "Joan Rivers' Cause of Death Was Lack of Oxygen to Her Brain." *Huffington Post*, October 16, 2014, http://www.huffingtonpost.com/2014/10/16/joan-rivers-cause-of-death_n_5998094.html.

Markham, N. I., and A. K. Lüi. "Diverticulitis of the Right Colon—Experience from Hong Kong." *Gut* 33 (1992): 547–49.

Mayo Clinic. "Dietary Fiber: Essential for a Healthy Diet," http://www.mayoclinic.org/healthy-lifestyle/nutrition-and-healthy-eating/in-depth/fiber/art-20043983.

Mayo Clinic Staff. "Gluten-Free Diet," http://www.mayoclinic.org/healthy-lifestyle/nutrition-and-healthy-eating/in-depth/gluten-free-diet/art-20048530.

McCartney, Anthony. "Michael Jackson Death Certificate Reflects Homicide Ruling." *USA Today*, September 1, 2009, http://usatoday30.usatoday.com/life/people/2009-09-01-jackson-death-certificate_N.htm.

McCombs, Jeffrey, Tara Matsuda, Ivy Tonnu-Mihara, et al. "The Risk of Long-Term Morbidity and Mortality in Patients with Chronic Hepatitis C: Results from an Analysis of Data from a Department of Veterans Affairs Clinical Registry." *JAMA Internal Medicine* 174, no. 2 (2014): 204–12.

McKenzie, Y. A., A. Adler, W. Anderson, et al. "British Dietetic Association Evidence-Based Guidelines for the Dietary Management of Irritable Bowel Syndrome in Adults." *Journal of Human Nutrition and Dietetics* 25 (2012): 260–74.

Medina, Jennifer. "Doctor Is Guilty in Michael Jackson's Death." *New York Times*, November 7, 2011, http://www.nytimes.com/2011/11/08/us/doctor-found-guilty-in-michael-jacksons-death.html?_r=0.

Methé, Barbara A., Karen E. Nelson, Mihai Pop, et al. "A Framework for Human Microbiome Research." *Nature* 486, no. 7402 (2012): 215–21.

Meyer, George W. "Endoscope Disinfection." *UpToDate*, last updated January 28, 2016, https://www.uptodate.com/contents/endoscope-disinfection?source=search_result&search=Endoscope+disinfect&selectedTitle=1%7E4.

Moran, Daniel. "Traveling and Eating Gluten-Free at Restaurants." *Celiac.com*, May 14, 2008, http://www.celiac.com/articles/21587/1/Traveling-and-Eating-Gluten-Free-at-Restaurants/Page1.html.

Morris, Arden M., Scott E. Regenbogen, Karin M. Hardiman, and Samantha Hendren. "Sigmoid Diverticulitis: A Systematic Review." *JAMA* 311, no. 3 (2014): 287–97.

Multi-Society Task Force. "Guidelines on Genetic Evaluation and Management of Lynch Syndrome: A Consensus Statement by the U.S. Multi-Society Task Force on Colorectal Cancer." *Gastrointestinal Endoscopy* 80, no. 2 (2014): 197–220.

National Cancer Institute. "Targeted Cancer Therapy," April 25, 2014, http://www.cancer.gov/about-cancer/treatment/types/targeted-therapies/targeted-therapies-fact-sheet.

National Cancer Institute. "Targeted Therapy." August 15, 2014, http://www.cancer.gov/about-cancer/treatment/types/targeted-therapies.

National Cancer Institute. "What Is Cancer?," last updated February 9, 2015, http://www.cancer.gov/about-cancer/understanding/what-is-cancer.

National Institute of Diabetes and Digestive and Kidney Diseases. "Definition and Facts for Irritable Bowel Syndrome," February 23, 2015, https://www.niddk.nih.gov/health-information/health-topics/digestive-diseases/irritable-bowel-syndrome/Pages/definition-facts.aspx.

National Institutes of Health. "Cancer Costs Projected to Reach at Least $158 Billion in 2020." January 12, 2011, https://www.nih.gov/news-events/news-releases/cancer-costs-projected-reach-least-158-billion-2020.

Navarro, Victor J., and M. Isabel Lucena. "Hepatotoxicity Induced by Herbal and Dietary Supplements." *Seminars in Liver Disease* 34, no. 2 (2014): 172–93.

Navarro, Victor J., Huiman Barnhart, Herbert L. Bonkovski, et al. "Liver Injury from Herbals and Dietary Supplements in the U.S. Drug-Induced Liver Injury Network." *Hepatology* 60, no. 4 (2014): 1399–1408.

Neff, Guy, Michael Jones, Taylor Broda, et al. "Durability of Rifaximin Response in Hepatic Encephalopathy." *Journal of Clinical Gastroenterology* 46, no. 2 (2012): 168–71.

Nielsen, Ole Haagen, and Mark Andrew Ainsworth. "Tumor Necrosis Factor Inhibitors for Inflammatory Bowel Disease." *New England Journal of Medicine* 369, no. 8 (2013): 754–62.

NIH Human Microbiome Project. "Microbiome Analyses," http://hmpdacc.org/micro_analysis/microbiome_analyses.php.

NIH Human Microbiome Project. "Overview—About the HMP," http://hmpdacc.org/micro_analysis/microbiome_analyses.php.

Nissen, Stephen E. "U.S. Dietary Guidelines: An Evidence-Free Zone." *Annals of Internal Medicine* 164, no. 8 (2016): 558–59.

Novick, David M. "Conquer Constipation: Why You're Backed Up and How to Fix It." *Fix* (blog), April 6, 2016, https://www.fix.com/blog/constipation-prevention-and-relief/.

Novick, David M. "Corticosteroids as Therapeutic Agents in Liver Diseases." *American Journal of Gastroenterology* 86, no. 1 (1991): 30–32.

Novick, David M., and Mary Jeanne Kreek. "Critical Issues in the Treatment of Hepatitis C Virus Infection in Methadone Maintenance Patients." *Addiction* 103, no. 6 (2008): 905–18.

Novick, David M., Roger W. Enlow, Alvin M. Gelb, et al. "Hepatic Cirrhosis in Young Adults: Association with Adolescent Onset of Alcohol and Parenteral Heroin Abuse." *Gut* 26, no. 1 (1985): 8–13.

Novick, Jane P., and David M. Novick. "Fight Ohio's Heroin Epidemic with the Most Effective Treatment." *Ohio Lawyer* 29, no. 6 (2015): 16–20.

Ong, Derrick K., Shaylyn B. Mitchell, Jacqueline S. Barrett, et al. "Manipulation of Dietary Short Chain Carbohydrates Alters the Pattern of Gas Production and Genesis of Symptoms in Irritable Bowel Syndrome." *Journal of Gastroenterology and Hepatology* 25 (2010): 1366–73.

Oxentenko, Amy S., and Joseph A. Murray. "Celiac Disease: Ten Things That Every Gastroenterologist Should Know." *Clinical Gastroenterology and Hepatology* 13, no. 8 (2015): 1396–1404.

Patel, D., M. J. W. McPhail, J. F. L. Cobbold, and S. D. Taylor-Robinson. "Hepatic Encephalopathy." *British Journal of Hospital Medicine* 73, no. 2 (2012): 79–85.

Patidar, Kavish R., and Jasmohan S. Bajaj. "Covert and Overt Hepatic Encephalopathy: Diagnosis and Management." *Clinical Gastroenterology and Hepatology* 13, no. 11 (2015): 2048–61.

Pemberton, John H. "Colonic Diverticulosis and Diverticular Disease: Epidemiology, Risk Factors, and Pathogenesis." *UpToDate*, last updated June 16, 2016, https://www.uptodate.com/contents/colonic-diverticulosis-and-diverticular-disease-epidemiology-risk-factors-and-pathogenesis?source=search_result&search=diverticulosis&selectedTitle=1%7E90.

Picarella, Dominic, Peter Hurlbut, James Rottman, et al. "Monoclonal Antibodies Specific for β_7 Integrin and Mucosal Addressin Cell Adhesion Molecules-1 (MAdCAM-1) Reduce Inflammation in the Colon of scid Mice Reconstituted with CD45RB[high] CD4+ T Cells." *Journal of Immunology* 158 (1997): 2099–2106.

Pohl, Heiko, Brenda Sirovich, and H. Gilbert Welch. "Esophageal Adenocarcinoma Incidence: Are We Reaching the Peak?" *Cancer Epidemiology, Biomarkers, & Prevention* 19, no. 6 (2010): 1468–70.

Poynard, Thierry, John McHutchison, Michael Manns, et al. "Impact of Pegylated Interferon and Ribavirin on Liver Fibrosis in Patients with Chronic Hepatitis C." *Gastroenterology* 122, no. 5 (2002): 1303–13.

Poynard, Thierry, Vlad Ratziu, Frédéric Charlotte, Zachary Goodman, John McHutchison, and Janice Albrecht. "Rates and Risk Factors of Liver Fibrosis Progression in Patients with Chronic Hepatitis C." *Journal of Hepatology* 34 (2001): 730–39.

Qaseem, Amir, Thomas D. Denberg, Robert H. Hopkins, et al. "Screening for Colorectal Cancer: A Guidance Statement from the American College of Physicians." *Annals of Internal Medicine* 156, no. 5 (2012): 378–86.

Quigley, Eammon M. M. "Leaky Gut: Concept or Clinical Entity." *Current Opinion in Gastroenterology* 32 (2016): 74–79.

Reau, Nancy. "HCV Testing and Linkage to Care: Expanded Access." *Clinical Liver Disease* 4, no. 2 (2014): 31–34. doi: 10.1002/cld.376.

Rex, Douglas K., David A. Johnson, Joseph C. Anderson, Phillip S. Schoenfeld, Carol A. Burke, and John M. Inadomi. "American College of Gastroenterology Guidelines for Colorectal Cancer Screening." *American Journal of Gastroenterology* 104, no. 3 (2009): 739–50.

Richter, Joel E., Gary W. Falk, and Michael F. Vaezi. "*Helicobacter pylori* and Gastroesophageal Reflux Disease: The Bug May Not Be All Bad." *American Journal of Gastroenterology* 93, no. 10 (1998): 1800–1802.

Rinella, Mary, and Michael Charlton. "The Globalization of Nonalcoholic Fatty Liver Disease: Prevalence and Impact on World Health." *Hepatology* 64, no. 1 (2016): 19–22.

Rizzo, Ellie. "What Really Happened to Joan Rivers? 7 Things to Know." September 19, 2014, http://www.beckersasc.com/asc-accreditation-and-patient-safety/what-really-happened-to-joan-rivers-7-things-to-know.html.

Rubenstein, Joel H., Hal Morgenstern, Henry Appelman, et al. "Prediction of Barrett's Esophagus among Men." *American Journal of Gastroenterology* 108, no. 3 (2013): 353–62.

Rutala, A., and David J. Weber. "Gastrointestinal Endoscopes: A Need to Shift from Disinfection to Sterilization?" *JAMA* 312, no. 14 (2014): 1405–1406.

Rutter, Matthew D., and Robert H. Riddell. "Colorectal Dysplasia in Inflammatory Bowel Disease: A Clinicopathological Perspective." *Clinical Gastroenterology and Hepatology* 12, no. 3 (2014): 359–67.

Sandborn, William J., Brian G. Feagan, Paul Rutgeerts, et al. "Vedolizumab as Induction and Maintenance for Crohn's Disease." *New England Journal of Medicine* 369, no. 8 (2013): 711–21.

Schaeffer, Juliann. "Gluten-Free Appetizers." *Today's Dietitian* 16, no. 12 (2014): 20, http://www.todaysdietitian.com/newarchives/120914p20.shtml.

Schoenfeld, Adam Jacob, and Deborah Grady. "Adverse Effects Associated with Proton Pump Inhibitors." *JAMA Internal Medicine* 176, no. 2 (2016): 172–74.

Shah, Shimul A., Gary A. Levy, Lesley D. Adcock, et al. "Adult-to-Adult Living Donor Liver Transplantation." *Canadian Journal of Gastroenterology* 20, no. 5 (2006): 339–43.

Shahedi, Kamyar, Garth Fuller, Roger Bolus, et al. "Long-Term Risk of Acute Diverticulitis among Patients with Incidental Diverticulosis Found during Colonoscopy." *Clinical Gastroenterology and Hepatology* 11, no. 12 (2013): 1609–13.

Shepherd, Sue, and Peter Gibson. *The Complete Low-FODMAP Diet.* New York: The Experiment, LLC, 2013.

Siegel, Rebecca, Carol DeSantis, and Ahmedin Jemal. "Colorectal Cancer Statistics, 2014." *CA: A Cancer Journal for Clinicians* 64 (2014): 104–17.

Singer, Elan. "Did Joan Rivers Die of VIP Syndrome?" *Forbes.com*, September 18, 2014, http://www.forbes.com/sites/realspin/2014/09/18/did-joan-rivers-die-of-vip-syndrome/.

Slavin, Joanne L. "Position of the American Dietetic Association: Health Implications of Dietary Fiber." *Journal of the American Dietetic Association* 108, no. 10 (2008): 1716–31.

Smith, Donald B., Jens Bukh, Carla Kuiken, et al. "Expanded Classification of Hepatitis C Virus into 7 Genotypes and 67 Subtypes: Updated Criteria and Genotype Assignment Web Resource." *Hepatology* 59, no. 1 (2014): 318–27.

Spechler, Stuart J., and Rhonda F. Souza. "Barrett's Esophagus." *New England Journal of Medicine* 371 (2014): 836–45.

Strate, Lisa A., Yan L. Liu, Sapna Syngal, Walid H. Aldoori, and Edward L. Giovannucci. "Nut, Corn, and Popcorn Consumption and the Incidence of Diverticular Disease." *Journal of the American Medical Association* 300, no. 8 (2008): 907–14.

Strum, Williamson B. "Colorectal Adenomas." *New England Journal of Medicine* 374, no. 11 (2016): 1065–75.

Substance Abuse and Mental Health Services Administration. "Sublingual and Transmucosal Buprenorphine for Opioid Use Disorder: Review and Update." *Advisory* 15, no. 1 (2016).

Sweetser, Seth, and Todd H. Baron. "Optimizing Bowel Cleansing for Colonoscopy." *Mayo Clinic Proceedings* 90, no. 4 (2015): 520–26.

Swift, Diana. "Sessile Serrated Adenomas: Abrupt Shift to Malignancy." *Medscape*, October 19, 2015, www.medscape.com/viewarticle/852899.

Szabo, Liz. "Why New Dietary Guidelines Matter." *USA Today*, January 7, 2016, http://www.usatoday.com/story/news/2016/01/07/why-new-dietary-guidelines-matter/77551410/.

Thalheimer, Judith C. "Gluten-Free Whole Grains—Choosing the Best Options While on a Gluten-Free Diet." *Today's Dietitian* 16, no. 10 (2014): 18, http://www.todaysdietitian.com/newarchives/100614p18.shtml.

United Network for Organ Sharing. "Living Donation," https://www.unos.org/donation/living-donation/.

United States Senate Committee on Finance. "Wyden-Grassley Sovaldi Investigation Finds Revenue-Driven Pricing Strategy behind $84,000 Hepatitis Drug." December 1, 2015, http://www.finance.senate.gov/ranking-members-news/wyden-grassley-sovaldi-investigation-finds-revenue-driven-pricing-strategy-behind-84-000-hepatitis-drug.

U.S. Department of Health and Human Services and U.S. Department of Agriculture. *2015–2020 Dietary Guidelines for Americans*. 8th Edition. Washington, DC: U.S. Department of Health and Human Services; December 2015, http://health.gov/dietaryguidelines/2015/.

van Hees, Frank, Dik F. Hebbema, Reinier G. Meester, Iris Lansdorp-Vogelaar, Marjolein van Ballegooijen, and Ann G. Zauber. "Should Colorectal Cancer Screening Be Considered in Elderly Persons without Previous Screening? A Cost-Effectiveness Analysis." *Annals of Internal Medicine* 160, no. 11 (2014): 750–59.

van Nood, Els, Anne Vrieze, Max Nieuwdorp, et al. "Duodenal Infusion of Donor Feces for Recurrent *Clostridium difficile*." *New England Journal of Medicine* 368, no. 5 (2013): 407–15.

Vermont Department of Health. "Living with C. Diff," http://healthvermont.gov/prevent/HAI/documents/Cdiff-2012.pdf.

Vierling, John M. "Legal Responsibilities of Physicians When They Diagnose Hepatic Encephalopathy." *Clinics in Liver Disease* 19 (2015): 577–89.

Vindigni, Stephen M., Timothy L. Zisman, David L. Suskind, et al. "The Intestinal Microbiome, Barrier Function, and Immune System in Inflammatory Bowel Disease: A Tripartite Pathophysiological Circuit with Implications for New Therapeutic Directions." *Therapeutic Advances in Gastroenterology* 9, no. 4 (2016): 606–25.

Voorhees, Corlyn, and Brittany Durgin. "Gluten-Free: The Truth Behind the Trend." *Worcester Magazine*, June 26, 2014, http://worcestermag.com/2014/06/26/gluten -free-truth-behind-trend/24723.

Vrieze, Anne, Els Van Nood, Frits Holleman, et al. "Transfer of Intestinal Microbiota from Lean Donors Increases Insulin Sensitivity in Individuals with Metabolic Syndrome." *Gastroenterology* 143, no. 4 (2012): 913–16.

Welch, H. Gilbert, and Douglas J. Robertson. "Colorectal Cancer on the Decline— Why Screening Can't Explain It All." *New England Journal of Medicine* 374, no. 17 (2016): 1605–1607.

Winawer, Sidney J., Ann G. Zauber, May Nah Ho, et al. "Prevention of Colorectal Cancer by Colonoscopic Polypectomy." *New England Journal of Medicine* 329, no. 27 (1993): 1977–81.

Wong, Florence. "Management of Ascites in Cirrhosis." *Journal of Gastroenterology and Hepatology* 27 (2012): 11–20.

Working Group IAP/APA Acute Pancreatitis Guidelines. "IAP/APA Evidence-Based Guidelines for the Management of Acute Pancreatitis." *Pancreatology* 13 (2013): e1–e15.

Xu, Jiaquan, Sherry L. Murphy, Kenneth D. Kocharnek, and Brigham A. Bastian. "Deaths: Final Data for 2013." *National Vital Statistics Reports* 64, no. 2 (2016): 1–119.

Yang, Daniel X., Cary P. Gross, Pamela R. Soulos, and James B. Yu. "Estimating the Magnitude of Colorectal Cancers Prevented during the Era of Screening." *Cancer* 120 (2014): 2893–2901.

Yang, Yu-Xiao, James D. Lewis, Solomon Epstein, and David C. Metz. "Long-Term Proton Pump Inhibitor Therapy and Risk of Hip Fracture." *JAMA* 296, no. 24 (2006): 2947–53.

Yeager, David. "Mapping the Gut Microbiome—An Ambitious Project That Could Lead to Better Gastrointestinal Health." *Today's Dietitian* 16, no. 9 (2014), http:// www.todaysdietitian.com/newarchives/090114p12.shtml.

Younossi, Zobair M., Aaron B. Koenig, Dinan Abdelatif, et al. "Global Epidemiology of Nonalcoholic Fatty Liver Disease—Meta-Analytic Assessment of Prevalence, Incidence, and Outcomes." *Hepatology* 64, no. 1 (2016): 73–84.

Zauber Ann G., Sidney J. Winawer, Michael J. O'Brien, et al. "Colonoscopic Polypectomy and Long-Term Prevention of Colonrectal-Cancer Deaths." *New England Journal of Medicine* 366, no. 8 (2012): 687–96.

For Further Reading

BOOKS

Elsagher, Brenda. *I'd Like to Buy a Bowel, Please*. Andover, MN, Expert Publishing, 2006.

Elsagher, Brenda. *It's in the Bag and under the Covers*. Andover, MN, Expert Publishing, 2011.

Enders, Giulia. *Gut: The Inside Story of Our Body's Most Underrated Organ*. Vancouver, Greystone Books, 2015.

Hauser, Stephen Crane, ed. *Mayo Clinic on Digestive Health*. Rochester, MN, Mayo Clinic, 2011.

Roach, Mary. *Gulp: Adventures on the Alimentary Canal*. New York, W.W. Norton & Company, 2013.

Shepherd, Sue, and Peter Gibson. *The Complete Low-FODMAP Diet*. New York, The Experiment, LLC, 2013.

Tauseef, Ali. *Crohn's and Colitis for Dummies*. New York, John Wiley & Sons, 2013.

WEBSITES

Academy of Nutrition and Dietetics	http://www.eatright.org
American Association for the Study of Liver Diseases	www.aasld.org
American Cancer Society	www.cancer.org
American College of Gastroenterology	www.gi.org
American Heart Association	www.heart.org
American Liver Foundation	http://www.liverfoundation.org
American Society for Gastrointestinal Endoscopy	www.asge.org
C Diff Foundation	www.cdifffoundation.org

Centers for Disease Control   www.cdc.gov
  and Prevention
Cleveland Clinic   http://my.clevelandclinic.org
Colon Cancer Alliance   http://www.ccalliance.org
Crohn's and Colitis Foundation   www.ccfa.org
  of America
Food and Drug Administration   http://www.fda.gov
Gluten-Free Living   http://www.glutenfreeliving.com
Human Microbiome Project   https://commonfund.nih.gov/hmp/index
International Agency for Research   http://www.iarc.fr
  on Cancer
Linus Pauling Institute, Oregon State http://lpi.oregonstate.edu/mic
  University
Mayo Clinic   http://www.mayoclinic.org
National Cancer Institute   www.cancer.gov
National Institute of Diabetes and   www.niddk.nih.gov
  Digestive and Kidney Diseases
Substance Abuse and Mental Health   http://www.samhsa.gov
  Services Administration
United Network for Organ Sharing   https://www.unos.org
UptoDate   https://www.uptodate.com/contents/
                                       table-of-contents/patient-information
U.S. Department of Agriculture   http://www.usda.gov/wps/portal/usda/
                                       usdahome
U.S. Department of Health and Human   http://www.hhs.gov
  Services

Partnership with GI Charities

The author intends to donate 10 percent of royalties received to charities that will benefit people with GI diseases.

Index

Page references for figures are italicized.

About the Author

David M. Novick, MD, is a board-certified gastroenterologist with extensive clinical and research experience. He is a Fellow in the American College of Physicians and the American Association for the Study of Liver Diseases. He is a clinical professor of internal medicine at Wright State University Boonshoft School of Medicine in Dayton, Ohio, and an adjunct faculty member at The Rockefeller University in New York City. Dr. Novick has written more than seventy medical publications. He is a 2014 Erma Bombeck Writing Competition award winner and is published in *Hippocampus Magazine*, Fix. com, and *Ohio Lawyer*. He is currently in private practice in gastroenterology with special interests in liver diseases and addiction medicine.